Neurosonography of the Pre-Term Neonate

Neurosonography of the Pre-Term Neonate

Edited by
Edward G. Grant

With Contributions by James D. Richardson,
Dieter Schellinger, Yolande F. Smith,
K.N. Siva Subramanian, and Edward G. Grant

With 97 Halftone Illustrations in 203 Parts

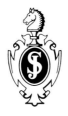

Springer-Verlag
New York Berlin Heidelberg Tokyo

Edward G. Grant, M.D.
Department of Radiology, Georgetown University Hospital, 3800 Reservoir Road, N.W., Washington, D.C. 20007, U.S.A.

Library of Congress Cataloging-in-Publication Data
Main entry under title:
Neurosonography of the pre-term neonate.
  Includes bibliographies and index.
  1. Brain—Diseases—Diagnosis. 2. Diagnosis,
Ultrasonic. 3. Cerebral anoxia—Complications and
sequelae. 4. Infants (Premature)—Diseases—Diagnosis.
I. Grant, Edward G.
[DNLM: 1. Brain Diseases—diagnosis. 2. Brain
Diseases—in infancy & childhood. 3. Infant,
Premature. 4. Ultrasonic Diagnosis. WS 340 N4948]
RJ290.5.N48 1986 618.92′807543 85-22180

Typeset by Bi-Comp, Inc., York, Pennsylvania.
Printed and bound by Halliday Lithograph, West Hanover, Massachusetts.
Printed in the United States of America.

9 8 7 6 5 4 3 2 1

ISBN 0-387-96219-0 Springer-Verlag New York Berlin Heidelberg Tokyo
ISBN 3-540-96219-0 Springer-Verlag Berlin Heidelberg New York Tokyo

To the technologists who taught me ultrasound
To John who taught me to write
And to my parents who taught me to enjoy life

Preface

Over a mere 5 years, neonatal cranial sonography has evolved from an obscure and largely experimental imaging possibility to the modality of preference in the examination of the young brain. The almost immediate acceptance of the ultrasound examination of the neonatal brain was based on a number of coincident factors, the most important of which was the emergence of a burgeoning population of premature neonates who were, for the first time, surviving beyond infancy. These delicate patients were beginning to withstand the rigors of extrauterine life when not fully prepared for it; pulmonary, cardiac, and infectious diseases no longer claimed most of them. With survival, a new specter reared its head: Would the eventual mental and neurologic status of these same children be worth the expense and time needed to bring them through their first months?

This issue became increasingly pressing as evidence mounted through the 1970s that very premature neonates were at a high risk for intracranial hemorrhage and posthemorrhagic complications. An imaging modality that could evaluate the premature brain was sorely needed. The CT scanner with its proven ability to diagnose intracranial hemorrhage was of little value in this regard. So too were static gray-scale or waterpath ultrasound units. These modalities all had the same limitation, lack of portability. As neonatal intensive care units proliferated, so did the technology that would soon allow cribside neonatal neuroimaging, the real-time sector scanner. This portable adaption of existing ultrasound technology became widely available at the ideal time as far as the neonatal intensive care nursery (ICN) was concerned.

In addition to portability, the sonographic sector scanner offered numerous other inherent advantages, enhancing its position as the preferred method of neonatal neuroimaging. The machines were relatively inexpensive, lessening the cost of individual examinations, and it was quickly realized how many cranial sonograms even a moderate-sized ICN could require per month. The scans were quickly and easily performed, and the smaller the patient (who could have imagined ANY patient weighing 500 g in 1975?), the better the resolution of the examination. If these advantages were not sufficient, we must also consider that as ultrasound is not a form of ionizing radiation, it may therefore be utilized repeatedly on the same patient without major concern for cellular damage.

In 1980, as promising early investigation catapulted the real-time sector scanner into the forefront, relatively little was known about the imaging of this unique group of patients. Today, 5 years later, we are still learning. The first sonographic description of periventricular leukomalacia (PVL) did not even occur until 1982. This particularly devastating intracranial process is intimately related to gestational immaturity. The pendulum, in fact, seems to be swinging, and it may be ischemia rather than hemorrhage that is the most important factor in the neurologic outcome of these children. Today, large numbers of once-premature children are reaching the preschool years. Although results are encouraging, our clinical follow-up must go much further, and detailed evaluation of sonographic data may eventually yield far more prognostic information than is possible at present.

This book is written to provide both the medical imager and the clinician with a detailed description of our present understanding of the premature brain as seen through the eyes of the sonogram. It is meant, however, to go beyond the mere imaging of the brain. This book is designed to tie pathophysiology, anatomy, and the all-important clinical follow-up data to the sonogram. The medical imager cannot operate in a vacuum. The sonographer needs to know why premature neonates suffer intracranial pathology so frequently and, more importantly, what his or her diagnoses mean. Circumstances will arise constantly in which the sonographer must advise the clinician, and occasionally even the parents themselves, about the meaning of certain, sometimes subtle, sonographic findings. Only the sonographer who is familiar with the reason a cerebral insult occurred and what it means prognostically can feel at ease in the ICN and act as a competent consultant rather than someone who merely takes pictures.

This book is divided into five basic parts. The first section, an introduction into scanning and normal anatomy, is meant to serve as a reference for those not entirely familiar with the subject; a portion on normal variants common to the immature brain ties this chapter into the main theme of the book. The reader is then acquainted with the pathophysiologic idiosyncrasies of the premature brain. According to Wigglesworth, the premature brain differs more from the brain of a term infant, just a few months more gestationally mature, than the brain of a term infant differs from that of an adult! With these basics in mind, the sonographic diagnosis of the two major forms of pathology unique to the premature brain is discussed in detail. I have tried to illustrate these sections liberally and to provide pathologic specimens for correlation when possible. Medical imaging is, after all, only a reflection of gross pathology.

Although we have described the sonography of the preterm brain, it is still incomplete without an adequate idea of what it means prognostically. A detailed discussion of our own experience and that of others in the field of clinical follow-up, therefore, constitutes the fifth and sixth chapters. An entire section is devoted almost exclusively to our own data on PVL. Ours is one of the largest post-ICN groups thus far studied; most other large series date back to the days before intensive-care nurseries. Regardless, the results are uniform; the diagnosis of PVL implies severe neurologic deficits in almost every case. We therefore contend that PVL in the preterm infant is the most important single neurodiagnosis that can be made. This is indeed a new concept, as germinal matrix hemorrhage has, for the most part, held center stage for over a decade. In closing, an attempt is made to keep ultrasound in proper perspective by presenting a neuroradiologist's overview. Although the sonogram may be the primary investigative tool in the examination of the preterm brain, appropriate use of other modalities (most notably CT scanning) can add a great deal of valuable information. Drawing from our own experience and relying heavily on others, we have attempted to assemble a detailed description of a subtle yet all important aspect of the premature patient.

Contents

Contributors

Edward G. Grant, MD
  Associate Professor of Radiology, Georgetown University, School of Medicine; Director Division of Ultrasound, Georgetown University Hospital, Washington, D.C., U.S.A.

James D. Richardson, MD
  Assistant Professor of Radiology, Georgetown University, School of Medicine, Washington, D.C. Presently Department of Radiology, MacGregor Medical Association, 8100 Greenbriar, Houston, Texas, U.S.A.

Dieter Schellinger, MD
  Professor of Radiology, Georgetown University School of Medicine, Director Division of Neuroradiology, Georgetown University Hospital, Washington, D.C., U.S.A.

Yolande F. Smith, MD
  Assistant Professor of Pediatrics, Georgetown University Hospital, Washington, D.C., U.S.A.

K. N. Siva Subramanian, MD
  Associate Professor of Pediatrics, Director of Neonatology, Georgetown University Hospital, Washington, D.C., U.S.A.

1
Scanning Techniques and Normal Anatomy

James D. Richardson
Edward G. Grant

This chapter begins with a discussion of the scanning modalities available for the evaluation of the premature neonatal cranium. Those modalities that are optimally employed in this regard will be differentiated from those that are not. We then undertake a brief discussion of scanning techniques, placing particular emphasis on the use of the sector scanner as it is the most widely used technology in the evaluation of the preterm brain. For those not already thoroughly familiar with such material, we present the normal sonographic anatomy of the infant cranium and its contents. Variations from the norm will be illustrated, with emphasis on the structural differences between term and preterm infants.

Background

Early clinical applications of ultrasound in the head were primarily confined to the A-mode display.[1] The major indication for A-mode scanning was the detection of intracranial midline shift, and while this was clinically useful, the limited nature of the information thus obtained did not generate much enthusiasm in the medical community. Early attempts at B-mode imaging in the neonatal head were not much more successful. The curved, uneven surface of the head makes transcranial contact scanning technically difficult, and the marked acoustic mismatch between the transducer and the skull generates considerable artifact in the nearfield, with consequent degradation of the image.

In an effort to overcome the problems associated with contact B-mode scanning, a number of investigators tried waterpath head scanning. A water-immersion technique was reported in 1965[2]; however, this method never gained widespread use, primarily because of the awkward positioning requirements for immersing the patient's head in a water tank. Based on the work of Garrett et al. in the development of the Octoson,[3] the use of a modified waterpath technique for the evaluation of intracranial pathology in infants was described by Haber et al. in 1980.[4] Although the field of view obtained with this scanning method is relatively large, enhancing anatomic orientation, resolution is limited by a relatively low-frequency transducer system and by the compounded sector-scanning technique. The high initial cost of such a system is also a major disadvantage[5]; however, the lack of portability restricts the use of this method to those infants stable enough to exist outside the protective environment of the isolette, effectively eliminating its application to the premature population.

In 1980, Ben-Ora et al. described the use of the anterior fontanelle as an acoustic window to the neonatal ventricular system.[6] Although the focus of their report was on the use of static B-mode contact scanners, they did point out that real-time imaging with a small transducer head could provide the same results in a shorter time. Several other investigators in rapid succession wrote of their experiences with real-time scanning through the anterior fontanelle,[7-9] and modern infant neurosonography became commonplace.

The anterior fontanelle provides a natural window to the infant brain, and is commonly

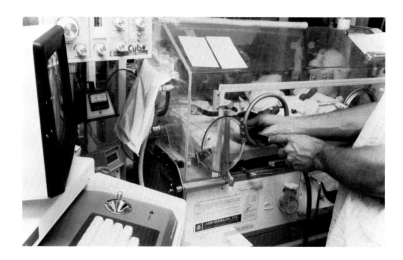

FIGURE 1-1. The portability of real-time ultrasound equipment allows the sonographer to perform examinations in the neonatal intensive care unit, thereby minimizing the risks of handling these very unstable infants. When necessary, babies can even be scanned without removing them from the protective environment of the isolette.

open through the first year of life. Its closure may be seen as early as 9 months, or as late as 30 months. In most infants closure is accomplished by 15 months, however.[10] The posterior fontanelle, in contrast, closes earlier, usually by 6 months of age.[11] There is considerable variation in the size of the anterior fontanelle among premature infants. Mechanical problems such as the molding of the skull bones and the occasional presence of a cephalhematoma can also diminish the effective size of this window. Iatrogenic impediments are also found: the veins in the infant's scalp are often utilized for intravenous access, thereby increasing the technical difficulty of the scan and degrading the quality of the image. In most infants, however, the anterior fontanelle provides easy access to the intracranial contents with excellent image quality, and the transfontanelle approach is now the accepted method of insonating the neonatal brain.

The real-time sector scanner is ideally suited to the relatively small window provided by the anterior fontanelle. Only a small contact area is required for imaging, and the field of view progressively widens as the distance from the transducer face increases, enabling visualization of the brain from one inner table to its opposite counterpart. In certain scanning situations, particularly obstetric examinations, the linear array real-time scanner has been employed with great success, its primary advantage over the sector scanner being its relatively larger field of view. However, due to the design of the liner array scanhead and the small con-

tact area provided by the anterior fontanelle, the field of view of the brain obtained in this manner is much smaller than that possible using the sector scanner. The smaller field of view and the mechanical coupling problems associated with the larger linear array scanheads have made the real-time sector scanner the scanhead of choice for cranial sonography in most medical centers. In an effort to overcome the difficulties associated with linear array scanners, Smith et al. devised a coupling apparatus to achieve better contact with the anterior fontanelle.[12] Even with this technical modification, use of the liner array scanner has not gained widespread acceptance.

Computed tomography (CT) was initially the "gold standard" for intracranial imaging in the neonate; with the advent of high-resolution real-time ultrasound, sonography now is employed as the primary imaging method in the neonatal cranium. The advantages of real-time sonography over CT include the lack of ionizing radiation, lower cost, and portability. As the incidence of intracranial pathology, particularly intracranial hemorrhage, is much higher in the premature infant than in the term neonate, the ultrasonographer must be primarily concerned with this population. The portable nature of real-time ultrasound therefore becomes a highly desirable feature, because of the instability of the premature neonate and the necessity for constant monitoring in the neonatal intensive care unit. Highly unstable infants can be examined without removing them from their isolettes, if necessary (Fig. 1-1).

FIGURE 1-2. A close-up view of the mechanical sector-scanner scanhead (**A**) demonstrates the relatively small contact area (*open arrow*) of this type of real-time ultrasound equipment. Within this scanhead are three separate ultrasound transducers, each of different frequency and focal length. By depressing the appropriate rotor element switch on the control panel of the machine (**B**), the operator may select the 3.0-, 5.0-, or 7.5-MHz transducer.

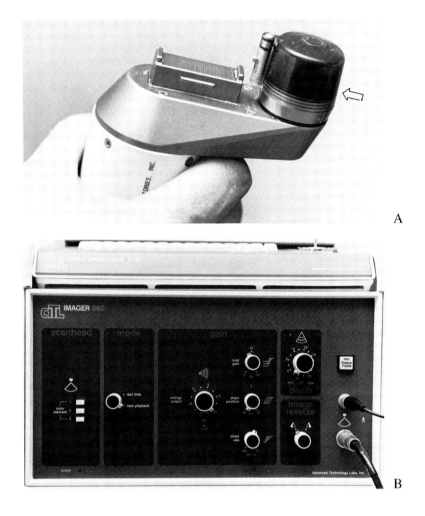

A

B

Scanning Techniques

The selection of transducer frequency and focal length should be optimized for the area of interest in each clinical examination. A 5.0-MHz transducer with a medium focal length is generally satisfactory for an overview of the entire brain in most infants; however, it is occasionally necessary to utilize a lower frequency in larger infants to ensure adequate penetration. The use of lower frequency transducers may be of particular value, for example, in follow-up studies, where the patient may be older and have a closing fontanelle. It is often helpful to scan with frequencies higher than 5.0 MHz to evaluate more superficial structures, including the areas of the germinal matrix, the periventricular white matter, and the extracerebral spaces. A 7.5-MHz transducer with a short focal length is ideal for this application, and high-resolution scanning in all preterm neonates is therefore strongly recommended. Because more than one transducer is often necessary in the evaluation of multiple infants in the nursery, a multifrequency scanhead offers the range of selection of frequency and focal length required without a great deal of cumbersome additional equipment (Fig. 1-2). Newer, computerized ultrasound units also offer advantages in this regard because they have variable focal zones.

The entire sonographic examination may be recorded on videotape, and in some centers this is the permanent archiving method. Hard copy of each examination is highly desirable, however, as serial scans are often obtained on these infants, and comparison is much easier when hard copy is available. A portable camera satisfies the need for film copy without compromising the portable nature of the equipment (Fig. 1-3).

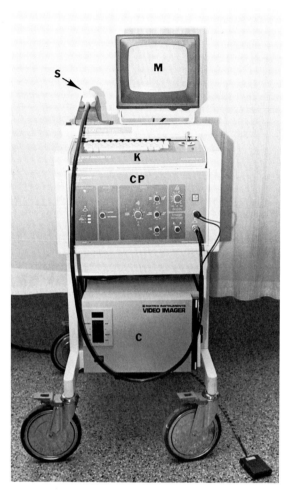

FIGURE 1-3. Complete portable real-time scanning apparatus. The ultrasound imaging equipment, including video monitor (*M*), scanhead (*S*), alphanumeric keyboard (*K*), and control panel (*CP*), is mounted on a lightweight wheeled cart. The cart can also accommodate a portable hard-copy camera (*C*) or, if desired, a videotape recorder (not shown).

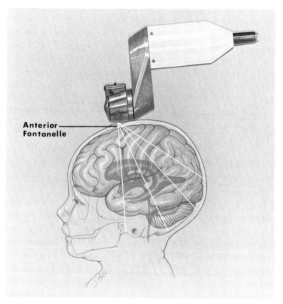

FIGURE 1-4. Orientation of scanhead on anterior fontanelle for coronal imaging. Scans in angled coronal, semiaxial, and axial planes are obtained by angling the scanner posteriorly. Note that with the scanhead placed on the infant's head in this fashion, the left–right orientation of the images is reversed from the conventional display. (Reprinted, with permission, from Grant E, et al. Real-time sonography of the neonatal and infant head. AJNR 1:487–492, 1980. Williams & Wilkins.)

The standard examination begins with the transducer oriented on the anterior fontanelle to produce images in the coronal plane, as depicted in Fig. 1-4. The scan plan is gradually angled posteriorly until a high axial plane is achieved, and the scanner is then turned on the fontanelle into the sagittal plane (Fig. 1-5). From the midline, the scanhead is gradually angled out laterally to produce angled parasagittal images until contact with the fontanelle is lost due to the steep angulation of the transducer. An infinite number of images can be generated with the real-time examination, and it is impor-

tant to sweep back and forth through the brain to gain an understanding of the three-dimensional anatomy in each infant. Certain images have become standardized, however, because of their optimal display of various important structures such as the ventricular system or the germinal matrix. These standardized images are then photographed with the hard-copy camera for the purposes of documentation and subsequent follow-up. The entire routine examination requires approximately 5–10 min.

It is occasionally useful to utilize scanning approaches other than that through the anterior fontanelle. Transcranial scanning through the coronal suture or the squamous portion of the temporal bone can demonstrate extracerebral fluid collections missed with the transfontanelle approach.[13] Although not as useful as the approach through the anterior fontanelle, the posterior fontanelle can also be used as a window to the neonatal brain. Occasionally, pathology in the occipital area or the posterior fossa may

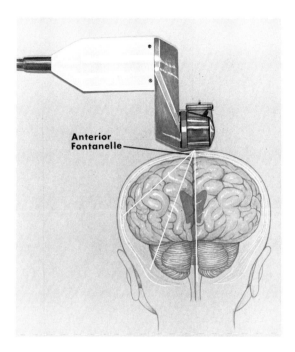

FIGURE 1-5. Orientation of scanhead on anterior fontanelle for sagittal imaging. Following scans in the midline, the scanner is gradually angled laterally to each side of the head to obtain the necessary angled parasagittal images. (Reprinted, with permission, from Grant E, et al. Real-time sonography of the neonatal and infant head. AJNR 1:487–492, 1980. Williams & Wilkins.)

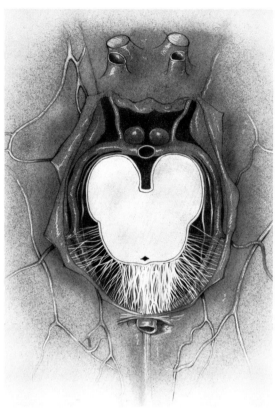

FIGURE 1-6. Horizontal section through midbrain in situ demonstrating interpeduncular, ambient, and quadrigeminal cisterns. Note fine trabeculae within subarachnoid space of quadrigeminal cistern. (Adapted from Key EAH, Retzius G. Studien in der Anatomie des Nervensystems und des Bingegewebes. Samson & Wallin, Stockholm, 1875.)

be demonstrated better with this approach. Infants with encephaloceles or high myelomeningoceles provide the sonographer with additional windows into the brain.

Normal Anatomy

Prior to a description of normal cross-sectional anatomy, a brief digression into the relative echogenicity of various intracranial structures is in order. The bones comprising the calvarium and the base of the skull are highly echogenic, as is the cerebellar vermis. The choroid plexus located in the roof of the third ventricle and in the bodies, atria, and temporal horns of the lateral ventricles also is of high-level echogenicity. In addition, various fissures and sulci, as well as the arterial vessels contained therein, appear as echogenic structures on sonographic images of the neonatal brain. Somewhat surprisingly, certain cisternal cerebrospinal fluid (CSF) spaces

appear echogenic: the interpeduncular cistern and the cistern of the quadrigeminal plate are two notable examples. The reason or reasons for the relatively high level of echogenicity of these fluid spaces is not known, but various theories have been put forward. Several authors have hypothesized that the echogenicity may be secondary to the pulsations of large vascular structures contained in these cisterns[14, 15]; others have postulated that the echogenicity may be secondary to the presence of numerous arachnoid trabeculae within these spaces[16] (Fig. 1-6).

The parenchyma of the brain stem and the cerebral and cerebellar hemispheres is of relatively low echogenicity, and in general is quite homogeneous. Exceptions to this rule include the basal ganglia, which demonstrate slightly

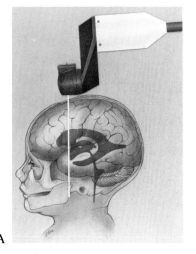

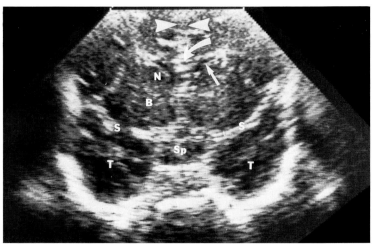

A

B

FIGURE 1-7. Coronal section at level of ICA bifurcation. *S* = Sylvian fissure, *T* = temporal lobe, *Sp* = sphenoid sinus, *arrow* = lateral ventricle, *curved arrow* = corpus callosum, *N* = caudate nucleus, *B* = basal ganglia (globus pallidus and putamen), *arrowheads* = interhemispheric fissure. (The authors wish to express appreciation to Dr. William Shuman and his associates for the use of the neonatal brain sections found in Figs 1-7 through 1-10, 1-12, 1-14, 1-16, and 1-17. Fig. 1-7 C reprinted, with permission, from Shuman W, Rogers J, Mack L, et al. Real-time sonographic sector scanning of the neonatal cranium: technique and normal anatomy. AJNR 2:349–356, 1981. Williams & Wilkins.)

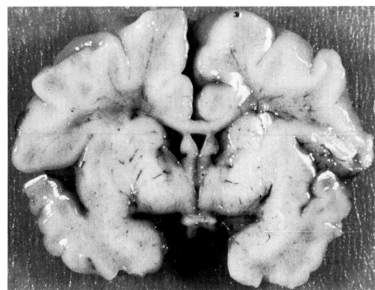

C

greater echogenicity than does the remainder of the cerebral parenchyma. Anechoic areas include the cisterna magna and small amounts of CSF in the lateral and fourth ventricles. The normal third ventricle is sufficiently small, and contains a relative paucity of CSF so that it does not appear anechoic but has an echogenicity similar to or slightly lower than that of the cerebrum. This is most likely on the basis of volume averaging of CSF and brain parenchyma.

An appreciation of normal anatomic structures is mandatory for the assessment of the infant brain for pathology. Much of what is now known of the sonographic anatomy of the brain is due to the excellent sonographic–anatomic–pathologic correlative work of numerous authors.[7–9, 14–20] Landmarks are provided by major vessels, the ventricular system, and various CSF spaces. This discussion of normal anatomy will follow the pattern set forth in the section on scanning techniques earlier in this chapter.

Section 1: Coronal at the Level of the Internal Carotid Artery Bifurcation

With the transducer oriented in the coronal plane, a section such as the one demonstrated in Fig. 1-7 can be obtained. The major landmark of this section is the origin of the middle cerebral artery bilaterally at the bifurcation of the supraclinoid internal carotid artery (ICA). The middle cerebral vessels can be seen extending laterally from the midline on both sides around the insula in the Sylvian fissures. During the real-time examination, the pulsations of the middle cerebral vessels can be easily identified. The Sylvian fissure so demarcated serves to separate the anterior temporal lobe from the insular cortex on each side. The nonaerated sphenoid sinuses can often be identified at this level as a somewhat rectangular structure of low echogenicity lying immediately inferior to the anterior clinoid processes.

The frontal horns of the lateral ventricles are tiny slitlike paramedian structures in the majority of normal neonates. Sometimes these fluid spaces can be identified as anechoic areas; at other times the small volume of CSF in this location cannot be resolved, and one merely identifies the specular boundary echoes of the superior and inferior borders of the anterior horns. Immediately cephalad to the superior boundary echo of the anterior horn, a small bright echo that can usually be identified extending laterally from the midline represents the sulcus of the corpus callosum. The area of brain parenchyma that lies between these two specular reflectors is the corpus callosum itself.

In general, the cerebral parenchyma has a homogeneous gray texture of relatively low echogenicity. However, the gray matter of the basal ganglia can often be identified as bilateral areas of slightly increased echogenicity relative to the adjacent white matter tracts. The head of the caudate nucleus represents the more superior aspect of the echo complex, lying immediately inferior to the anterior horn of the lateral ventricle on each side. The more inferior portion of the basal ganglia echo complex at this level is composed of the putamen and globus pallidus.

A bright midline echo is usually identified extending inferiorly from the top of the sector image to the region of the corpus callosum; this represents the junction of the medial surfaces of the frontal cortex bilaterally with the falx cerebri in the interhemispheric fissure. Normally, the falx cannot be distinguished from the adjacent frontal cortex, and an anechoic CSF space is not identified at this level. In the presence of extracerebral fluid in this location, however, the falx can be outlined as a distinct midline structure that is clearly separated from the medial surface of the frontal lobes on each side.

Section 2: Coronal at the Level of the Interpeduncular Cistern

If the transducer is moved slightly posteriorly on the anterior fontanelle from the position at which Section 1 is taken, the section illustrated in Fig. 1-8 comes into view. The echogenic interpeduncular cistern serves as the landmark for this section. Within the cistern, the pulsations of the basilar artery can be noted during the real-time exam. Inferiorly, the belly of the pons and the proximal portion of the medulla are visualized as homogeneous structures having intermediate echogenicity. The brightly echogenic curving arcs on either side of the echogenic interpeduncular cistern are composites of the circular sulci, which separate the medial aspect of the temporal lobes from the adjacent brain stem, and the choroidal fissures, from which the choroid plexus invaginates into the adjacent temporal horns.

The hypoechoic structures lying between the interpeduncular cistern and the choroidal fissure on either side are the cerebral peduncles. The middle cerebral artery branches can be visualized as echogenic Y-shaped bands projecting medially from the lateral cerebral cortex bilaterally. The anterior horns of the lateral ventricles and the corpus callosum appear as described in Section 1. The distinction between basal ganglia and the adjacent white matter of the internal capsule is not as pronounced as in the previous section; often these areas appear of uniform low-level echogenicity. The third ventricle is present in this section; however, the transverse diameter of the third ventricle is so small that an anechoic CSF space is not seen. If the ventricle is dilated, however, it can be easily visualized in this plane.

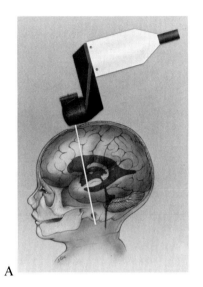

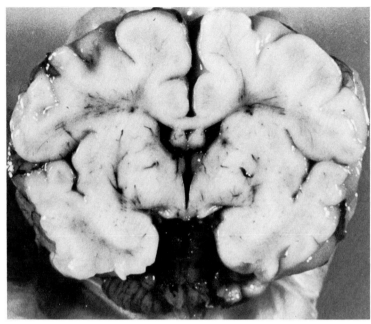

C

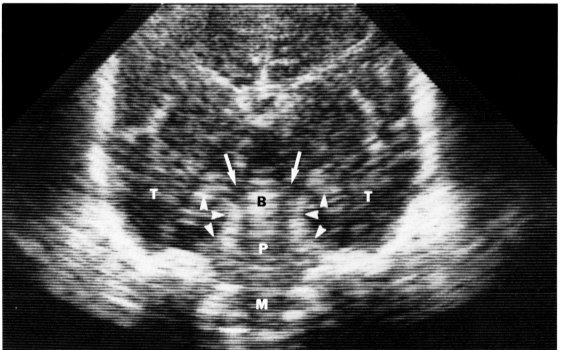

B

FIGURE 1-8. Coronal section at level of interpeduncular cistern. *B* = interpeduncular cistern/basilar artery, *P* = pons, *M* = medulla oblongata. *Arrowheads* point to echogenic arcs which are composites of the choroidal fissure (*upper arrowheads*), the circular sulci (*middle arrowheads*) and the medial portion of the tentorium cerebelli (*lower arrowheads*). *Arrows* = cerebral peduncles, *T* = temporal lobes. (Fig. 1-8 C reprinted, with permission, from Shuman W, Rogers J, Mack L, et al. Real-time sonographic sector scanning of the neonatal cranium: technique and normal anatomy. AJNR 2:349–356, 1981. Williams & Wilkins.)

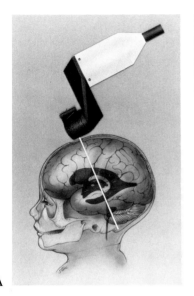

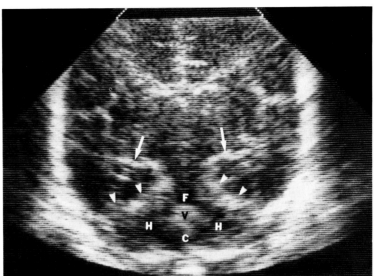

FIGURE 1-9. Angled coronal section at level of fourth ventricle. *F* = Fourth ventricle, *V* = inferior vermis, *C* = cisterna magna. *Arrowheads* = tentorium cerebelli, *arrows* = choroidal fissures, *H* = cerebellar hemispheres. (Fig. 1-9 C reprinted, with permission, from Shuman W, Rogers J, Mack L, et al. Real-time sonographic sector scanning of the neonatal cranium: technique and normal anatomy. AJNR 2:349–356, 1981. Williams & Wilkins.)

Section 3: Angled Coronal at the Level of the Fourth Ventricle

Angling the transducer further posteriorly brings the examiner into the plane of Fig. 1-9. The landmark of this section, the fourth ventricle, can be seen as a rectangular or rhomboid-shaped anechoic space in the midline inferiorly. Posterior and inferior to the fourth ventricle is a linear band of echogenicity that represents a combination of through-transmission from the fluid in the ventricle plus the inferior aspect of the cerebellar vermis. The cisterna magna may be seen at this level as an anechoic area in the midline far inferiorly, interposed between the inferior vermis and the occipital bone. The choroidal fissures extend inferolaterally at this level into the two leaves of the tentorium cere-

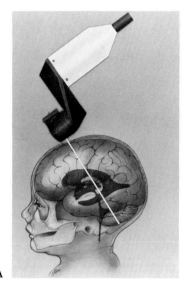

A

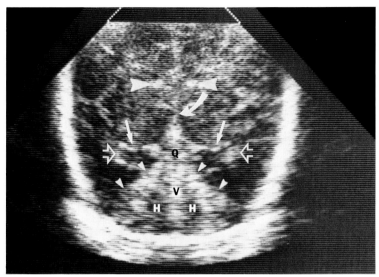

B

FIGURE 1-10. Semiaxial section at level of quadrigeminal plate cistern. *Q* = quadrigeminal plate cistern, *curved arrow* = tela choroidea, *arrows* = choroidal fissures, *small arrowheads* = tentorium, *open arrows* = inferior portion of the glomus of choroid plexus, *H* = cerebellar hemispheres, *V* = superior vermis, *large arrowheads* = choroid plexus in bodies of lateral ventricles. (Fig. 1-10 C reprinted, with permission, from Shuman W, Rogers J, Mack L, et al. Real-time sonographic sector scanning of the neonatal cranium: technique and normal anatomy. AJNR 2:349–356, 1981. Williams & Wilkins.)

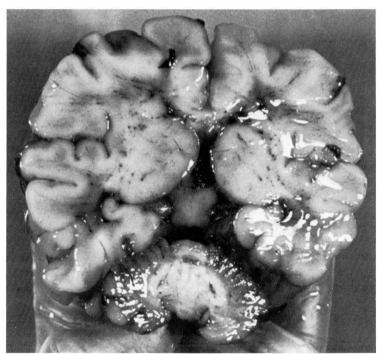

C

belli. The hypoechoic areas lateral to the echogenic midline vermis beneath the tentorium represent the cerebellar hemispheres. More superficially, the Sylvian fissures appear as in the previous section. Portions of the bodies of the lateral ventricles now appear as anechoic paramedian structures. Although the third ventricle and the aqueduct of Sylvius usually lie in this plane of section, these structures cannot be resolved and visualized in the absence of hydrocephalus.

Section 4: Semiaxial at the Level of the Quadrigeminal Plate Cistern

Further posterior angulation of the scanner will produce an image in a semiaxial plane as depicted in Fig. 1-10. The identifying landmark of

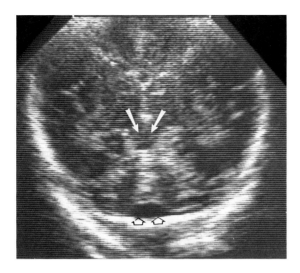

FIGURE 1-11. Semiaxial scan through quadrigeminal plate. Hypoechoic corpora quadrigemina (*arrows*) project into the echogenic quadrigeminal cistern. Note also cisterna magna (*open arrows*), easily seen posterior and inferior to cerebellar vermis in this infant.

this section is a brightly echogenic starshaped figure; the "star" is a composite of several structures.[15, 16] Its central portion represents the echogenic cistern of the quadrigeminal plate; often, the superior and inferior colliculi, which comprise the quadrigeminal plate, can be visualized as a hypoechoic rectangular area within the echogenic cistern in the central portion of the star (Fig. 1-11). The anterior point of the star is the tela choridea of the third ventricle, containing echogenic choroid plexus as well as several large veins. The lateral limbs or "arms" of the star represent the choroidal fissures, here pointing to the most inferior portions of the glomus of the choroid plexus of the lateral ventricles (Fig. 1-12). The "legs" of the star are the leaves of the cerebellar tentorium, delimiting the posterior fossa and separating it from the adjacent temporal cortex. The echogenic structure in the midline in the posterior fossa is the cerebellar vermis, with the two cerebellar hemispheres seen as relatively hypoechoic areas to either side of the midline. The cisterna magna may also be visible at this level (Fig. 1-11). The Sylvian fissures and bodies of the lateral ventricles appear as in the previous section.

Section 5: Axial at the Level of the Glomus of the Choroid Plexus in the Lateral Ventricles

By angling the scanner further posterior and superior from the previous level, an image is obtained as depicted in Fig. 1-12. Here, the glomus of the choroid plexus in the atrium or trigone of each lateral ventricle serves as the identifying landmark. The choroid is, as always, brightly echogenic, and should demonstrate smooth margins. Although the lateral ventricles can appear asymmetrical in this section in normal infants,[21] any large disparity in size should alert the sonographer to possible pathology. Small amounts of anechoic CSF are usually visualized surrounding the choroid plexus bilaterally. Lateral to the ventricles on each side, the normal periventricular echogenicity should be noted; this normal echogenicity is never as bright as the adjacent choroid plexus. A horizontally oriented echogenic line can often be seen extending laterally from the midline between the bodies of the lateral ventricles; this line demarcates the splenium of the corpus callosum. The interhemispheric fissure is variably seen in this section as a vertically oriented echogenic line in the midline. At this level, in the term infant, the echoes of the Sylvian fissures are joined by various superficial cortical sulci, manifested by echogenic lines extending medially from the inner tables of the skull bilaterally.

Section 6: Axial above the Level of the Lateral Ventricles

Extreme posterior and cephalad angulation of the transducer brings the sonographer into the plane of Fig. 1-13. This is the most cephalad image that can usually be obtained using contact scanning through the anterior fontanelle. There are no ventricular or cisternal landmarks in this section; rather, the interhemispheric fissure containing the falx cerebri serves as the identifying structure, running longitudinally in the midline from anterior to posterior. Various superficial cortical sulci are visible as in the previous section, extending medially from the lateral margins of the superficial brain cortex as well as extending laterally from the midline.

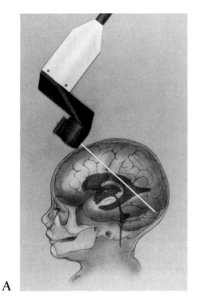

A

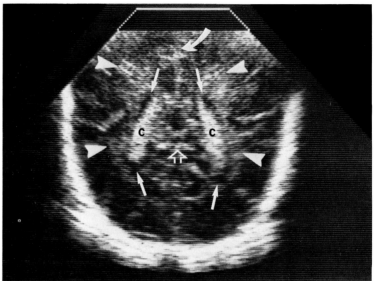

B

FIGURE 1-12. Axial scan at level
of glomus of choroid plexus. *C* =
choroid plexus, *open arrow* =
splenium of corpus callosum,
curved arrow = interhemispheric
fissure. *Arrows* point to CSF in
lateral ventricles and *arrowheads*
delineate the normal periventricular echogenic halo. (Fig. 1-12
C reprinted, with permission,
from Shuman W, Rogers J, Mack
L, et al. Real-time sonographic
sector scanning of the neonatal
cranium: technique and normal
anatomy. AJNR 2:349–356,
1981. Williams & Wilkins.)

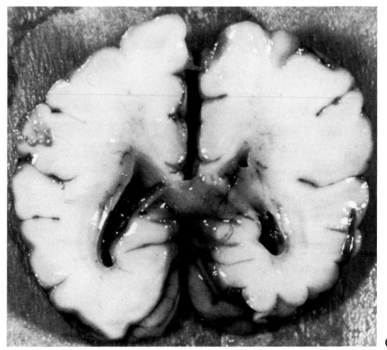

C

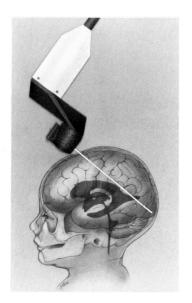

A

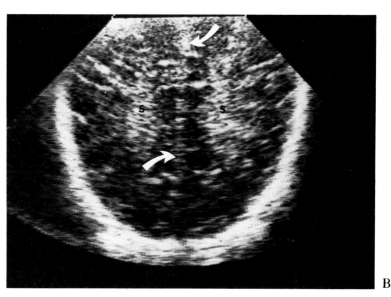

B

FIGURE 1-13. Axial scan above level of lateral ventricles. *Curved arrows* = interhemispheric fissure, *S* = centrum semiovale.

The white matter cephalad to the bodies of the lateral ventricles, which is a large portion of the brain visible in this section, appears as areas of irregularly shaped echogenicity on either side of the midline. There is considerable variability in the size, shape, and degree of echogenicity of these ares; however, the sonographer should be aware of this normal periventricular "halo"[22] to avoid confusing it with certain pathologic states that are described later.

Section 7: Midline Sagittal

Turning the scanhead 90° on the fontanelle from the coronal plane prepares the examiner for sagittal and parasagittal imaging. When the transducer is brought into the midline, the image depicted in Fig. 1-14 is produced. The posterior landmark in this section is the highly echogenic cerebellar vermis, a somewhat oval structure indented anteriorly by a small cleft, the fourth ventricle. Extending anterosuperiorly from the vermis is an echogenic band that represents the quadrigeminal plate cistern; immediately anterior and inferior to the midportion of the cistern are the hypoechoic corpora quadrigemina, arising from the doral aspect of the brain stem. Continuing anteriorly, the band of echogenicity curves inferiorly into the tela

choroidea of the third ventricle, containing its echogenic choroid plexus. Immediately anterior and superior to the tela choroidea of the third ventricle is the septum pellucidum. Surrounding the septum pellucidum and extending posteriorly is the corpus callosum, which is demarcated superiorly by an echogenic arc representing the sulcus of the corpus callosum. Several other echogenic arcs can be identified parallel and cephalad to the sulcus of the corpus callosum, which are various cerebral sulci containing branches of the anterior cerebral artery. These arterial branches demonstrate characteristic pulsations during the real-time examination.

Between the echogenic clivus and the quadrigeminal plate cistern is a small area of bright echogenicity, the interpeduncular cistern. As pointed out in the discussion of Section 2, the distal aspect of the basilar artery is contained in this cistern, and pulsations can be noted during the real-time exam. The brain stem lies posterior and inferior to the interpeduncular cistern, its low-level echogenicity contrasted by the high-level echoes of the clivus and pontine cistern anteriorly and the vermis posteriorly. Rarely, the normal-sized third ventricle can be distinguished as a discrete structure in this image; instead of appearing anechoic, it is only

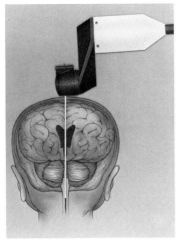

A

FIGURE 1-14. Midline sagittal scan. *V* = cerebellar vermis, *small arrow* = fourth ventricle, *Q* = corpora quadrigemina, *small arrowhead* = quadrigeminal plate cistern, *open arrows* = tela choroidea, *S* = cavum septi pellucidi, *large arrowheads* = corpus callosum, *curved arrows* = cerebral sulci containing branches of the anterior cerebral/ pericallosal artery system, *I* = interpeduncular cistern/basilar artery, *B* = belly of pons, *P* = pons, *M* = medulla oblongata, *C* = cisterna magna, *T* = third ventricle. (Fig. 1-14 C reprinted, with permission, from Shuman W, Rogers J, Mack L, et al. Real-time sonographic sector scanning of the neonatal cranium: technique and normal anatomy. AJNR 2:349–356, 1981. Williams & Wilkins.)

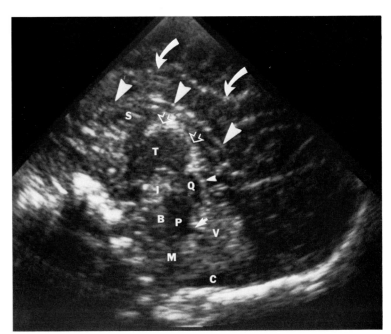

B

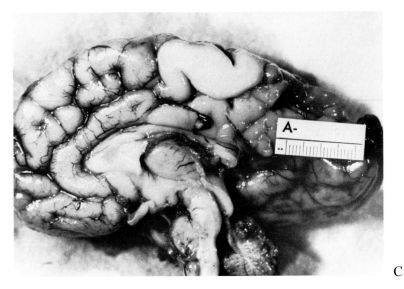

C

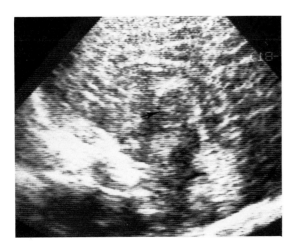

FIGURE 1-15. Midline sagittal scan. Small echogenic focus (*arrow*) inferior to arc of tela choroidea of third ventricle represents the massa intermedia. This structure is infrequently visualized in the absence of hydrocephalus.

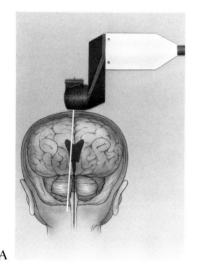

A

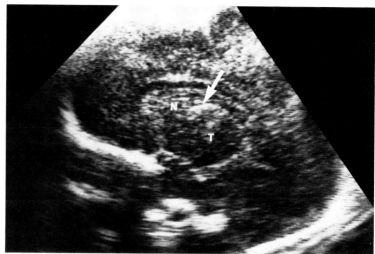

B

FIGURE 1-16. Angled parasagittal scan at level of caudothalamic groove. *N* = caudate nucleus, *T* = thalamus, *arrow* = caudothalamic groove. (Fig. 1-16 C reprinted, with permission, from Shuman W, Rogers J, Mack L, et al. Real-time sonographic sector scanning of the neonatal cranium: technique and normal anatomy. AJNR 2:349–356, 1981. Williams & Wilkins.)

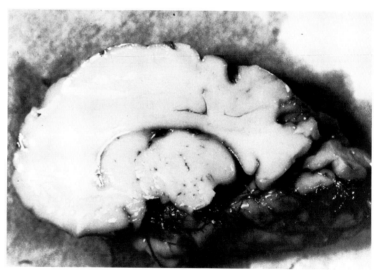

C

slightly lower in echogenicity than the cerebrum, most likely secondary to its small transverse diameter. Occasionally, the massa intermedia can be visualized as a small echogenic focus lying inferior to the arc of the tela choroidea of the third ventricle (Fig. 1-15). Visualization of the massa intermedia is facilitated by the presence of hydrocephalus involving the third ventricle.

Section 8: Angled Parasagittal at the Level of the Caudothalamic Groove

Very slight lateral angulation of the transducer from the midline sagittal plane will bring the plane of Fig. 1-16 into view. This particular plane is often best demonstrated with a degree of scanning obliquity; the anterior portion lies somewhat more medial than the posterior. The landmark of this section is the caudothalamic groove, a brightly echogenic arc separating the head of the caudate nucleus anteriorly from thalamus posteriorly. Identification of this scan plane is important in the evaluation of the preterm infant, as the residual germinal matrix tissue in the majority of gestationally immature neonates lies immediately anterior to this echogenic arc.[23] Portions of the frontal horn and body of the lateral ventricle are noted superiorly. *The caudate nucleus again demonstrates a slightly greater echogenicity than does the thalamus.*

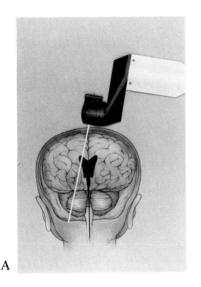

A

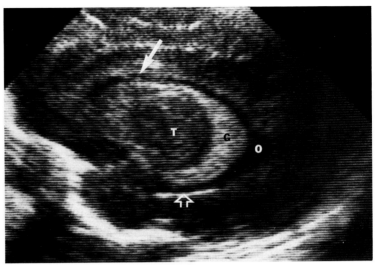

B

FIGURE 1-17. Angled parasagittal
scan at level of lateral ventricle.
G = glomus of choroid plexus,
arrow = frontal horn, *O* = occipital horn, *open arrow* = temporal
horn of lateral ventricle, *T* =
thalamus. (Fig. 1-17 C reprinted,
with permission, from Shuman
W, Rogers J, Mack L, et al. Real-
time sonographic sector scanning
of the neonatal cranium: technique and normal anatomy.
AJNR 2:349–356, 1981. Williams
& Wilkins.)

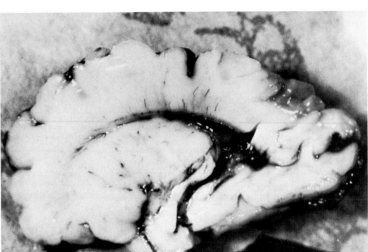

C

Section 9: Angled Parasagittal at the Level of the Lateral Ventricle

A small amount of lateral movement of the scanner on the fontanelle coupled with further lateral angulation and posterior divergence brings the plane of the body and atrium of the lateral ventricle into view (Fig. 1-17). The visualized portions of the lateral ventricle in this section describe a C-shaped curvature (here reversed). The highly echogenic glomus of the choroid plexus in the atrium of the lateral ventricle serves as a landmark. The choroid extends anteriorly into the body of the lateral ventricle, and then dives medially through the foramen of Monro into the third ventricle. It is important to note that the choroid does not ex-

tend into the frontal horn. Any echogenicity in this region (anterior to the level of the foramen of Monro) should be carefully evaluated to rule out the presence of intraventricular hemorrhage. In general, the contour of the choroid plexus is smooth, and any irregularity or "lumpiness" should raise the suspicion of adjacent intraventricular hemorrhage.

A variable amount of CSF may be seen in the lateral ventricle as an anechoic rim about the superior aspect of the choroid plexus. In many neonates, it is difficult to discern any anechoic fluid in this section because of the relatively large size of the choroid plexus. Unless the lateral ventricle is dilated, it may be difficult to bring the atrium of the lateral ventricle with its three extensions, the frontal, occipital, and

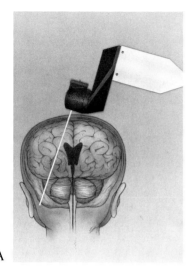
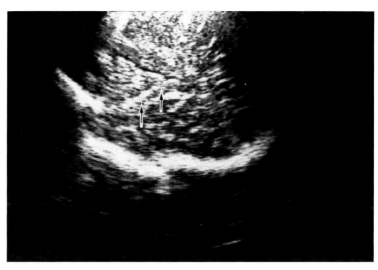

A   B

FIGURE 1-18. Angled parasagittal scan lateral to temporal horn of lateral ventricle. *Arrows* point to Sylvian fissure. Convolutions emanating from it indicate this section is from a gestationally mature neonate. Compare this with Figure 1-22.

temporal horns, into the same plane of section. The entirety of the lateral ventricle may be evaluated during the real-time examination, however, by sweeping the scanner through the ventricular system from medial to lateral and back again. The hypoechoic area within the curve described by the glomus of the choroid plexus is the thalamus. Various portions of the frontal, parietal, occipital, and temporal lobes are visible in this section about the arc of the lateral ventricle.

Section 10: Angled Parasagittal Lateral to the Temporal Horn

Further lateral angulation of the scanner will produce a section lateral to the temporal horn of the lateral ventricle, as shown in Fig. 1-18. As in Section 6, there is no major vascular, cisternal, or ventricular landmark for this section; rather, the obliquely oriented echoes delineating the Sylvian fissure serve as a reference point. Depending on the gestational age of the infant, a variable number of small linear and curvilinear echoes can be seen scattered throughout this section that represent various sulci about the convolutions of the cerebrum. As the number of cerebral convolutions increases with brain maturation,[24] it follows that the number of convolutional echoes seen in this

section varies with the gestational age. It usually is not possible to obtain images further lateral to this section, due to loss of contact with the fontanelle because of the steep angulation required for such an image.

Normal Variants

After a discussion of normal anatomy, it is appropriate to emphasize certain commonly encountered variants, which, unless appreciated as normal findings, may be easily confused with pathology. Most of these normal variants are typically associated with gestational immaturity. Brief note will also be made of several scanning artifacts that may be seen during the examination of the neonatal brain.

Cavum Septi Pellucidi and Cavum Vergae

Two anatomic variants that are often encountered in the premature population are the cavum septi pellucidi and the cavum vergae. These two midline fluid spaces are bounded superiorly by the corpus callosum and inferiorly by the two arches of the fornix. The two halves of the fornix, one located in each cerebral hemisphere, approach each other closely in the mid-

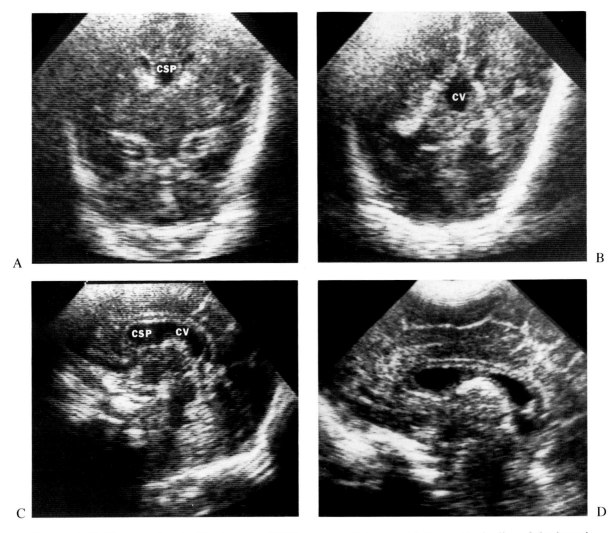

FIGURE 1-19. Cava septi pelucidi et vergae (*CSP*, cavum septi pellucidi; *CV*, cavum vergae.) Angled coronal scan (**A**) demonstrates the cystic cavum septi pellucidi in its normal location in the midline between the anterior horns of the lateral ventricles. Semiaxial scan (**B**) shows the more posterior cavum vergae interposed between the bodies of the lateral ventricles. In midline sagittal image (**C**), the relationship of these two structures is shown. (**D**) Fluid space inferior to cavum vergae, possibly representing a large, septated cavum vergae.

line at the apex of the curvature of each arc, and then diverge slightly laterally as these arcs continue anteriorly and posteriorly. The point at which they approach each other in the midline serves to separate the cavum septi pellucidi anteriorly from the cavum vergae posteriorly. These two cavi are in free communication with each other,[11, 25] but controversy exists over the source of the fluid contained in each. A pathologic study of these cavities published in 1969[25] contends that normally they do not communicate with either the ventricular or cisternal CSF spaces of the brain; however, communication with the ventricular system seems apparent at pneumoencephalography.[11] It is normal to encounter these two fluid spaces in the fetus; however, closure of the cavum vergae begins in utero at about 6 months of gestation. The closure progresses from posterior to anterior, and just prior to term, the cavum septi pellucidi has begun to close.[25] It is therefore not surprising to note the presence of a cavum septi pellucidi in 100% of premature neonates. The incidence progressively diminishes with advancing age, so that after approximately 2 months of postpartum life, the cavum septi pellucidi is no longer present in most infants.[25]

The cavum septi pellucidi may vary widely in size, ranging from a tiny slitlike space to a cavity considerably larger than the neighboring anterior horns of the lateral ventricles. There do not appear to be any data specifically linking the size of the cavum with the presence of central nervous system (CNS) symptoms; however, if the cavum becomes large enough to cause obstruction to ventricular flow, the symptoms and signs of hydrocephalus will ensue.[25]

In neonatal sonography, the cavum septi pellucidi appears as a well-defined cystic region in coronal scans interposed between the anterior horns of the lateral ventricles (Fig. 1-19 A). The cavum vergae is well visualized at a more posterior level on an angled coronal or semiaxial scan, interposed between the bodies and trigones of the lateral ventricles (Fig. 1-19 B). These continuous cystic structures are seen well in the midline sagittal scan (Fig. 1-19 C). An infrequently encountered but apparently related variant is a cystic space located inferior to the cavum vergae (Fig. 1-19 D). This space seems separated from the cavum vergae by a prominent septation that is clearly visualized in both the sagittal and angled coronal sections. This cystic space may represent a large, posterior extension of the cavum vergae with an internal membrane. Although one might be tempted to call this the cavum veli interpositi, its shape on angled coronal sections is not typical of that structure. We know of no anatomic study that has definitely described this cystic space, but we have never identified it in a neonate who did not have both a prominent cavum septi pellucidi and cavum vergae in addition. Regardless of its actual name, the sonographer should consider this anechoic structure another of the normal variants associated with prematurity.

Ventricular System

While the human body is highly symmetrical, slight degrees of asymmetry between the left and right sides of the body are universal. Not only does this apply to external features, but the two hemispheres of the normal brain also participate in this left–right asymmetry. In a recent study,[21] mild degrees of asymmetry in size between the two lateral ventricles were identified with sonography in infants with no known cerebral pathology. In most infants demonstrating lateral ventricular asymmetry, the left lateral ventricle was larger than the right. It therefore appears likely that mild degrees of asymmetry in the size of the two lateral ventricles can be normal. There are no absolute criteria to distinguish cases of normal asymmetry from pathologic ventricular dilatation. The greater the degree of asymmetry, however, the more the sonographer should look for additional evidence of pathology. In borderline cases, serial examinations may be the only way to establish the significance of the findings.

Similarly, there is a high degree of variability in the presence and relative size of the occipital horns of the two lateral ventricles. In fact, asymmetry is the rule rather than the exception.[26] This variation in the occipital horn includes bilateral absence, unilateral absence, and both symmetry and asymmetry in size when both horns are present (Fig. 1-20).

In addition to the asymmetries mentioned previously, the entire ventricular system should be viewed within the context of the developmental stage of the infant. Because of differen-

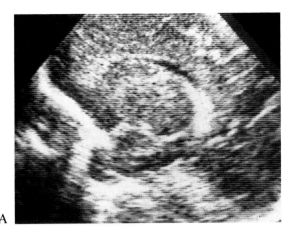 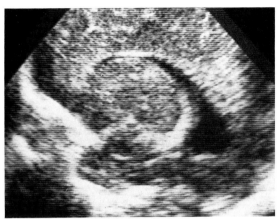

A   B

FIGURE 1-20. Angled parasagittal scans through the bodies and occipital horns of right (**A**) and left (**B**) lateral ventricles in same infant. Note asymmetry in size of occipital horns. No evidence of intraventricu- lar hemorrhage or other pathology was demon- strated, and serial scans in this infant showed no evidence of progression in the size of the left lateral ventricle.

tial growth rates, the relative size of the lateral ventricles and the cerebral cortex changes dur- ing development: as the fetus matures, the size of the lateral ventricle diminishes relative to the size of the adjacent cortex. Hence, the ventric- ular system appears relatively larger in the pre- term than in the term infant.[26] Neurosono- graphy of the term infant usually demonstrates the anterior horns of the lateral ventricles as tiny slitlike areas of echogenicity in the coronal plane. In the premature infant, however, the anterior horns and the remainder of the ventric- ular system may appear larger relative to the overall size of the cerebral mantle. These dis- tinctions should be borne in mind when evaluat- ing the neonatal brain for the presence of hydro- cephalus.

Finally, one particular source of confusion deserves inclusion in this discussion on the nor- mal appearance of the lateral ventricles. The calcarine fissure often produces a prominent impression on the medial wall of the lateral ven- tricle. This impression may, in fact, simulate a mass or even clot within the ventricle in parasa- gittal sections. Slight lateral angulation of the sound beam will usually solve this diagnostic dilemma by bringing the main portion of the trigone into view and confirming that the appar- ent mass is no more than the normal curve of the medial wall of the lateral ventricle around the calcarine fissure.

Cisterna Magna

The size of the cisterna magna is variable in the normal neonatal population. According to Goodwin and Quisling, the midsagittal height of this cistern ranges from 3 to 8 mm in normal infants, with a mean value of 4.5 mm.[27] Various types of posterior fossa pathology have been shown to abnormally increase the size of the cisterna magna, and in cases of the Arnold– Chiari type II malformation, the sonographi- cally visualized cisterna magna is small and may be totally obliterated by the downward dis- placement of the cerebellum. An appreciation of the normal range of size for this cistern there- fore becomes important. For examples of the variations in the size of the normal cisterna magna, the reader is referred to Figs. 1-9, 1-10, 1-11, 1-14, 1-15, and 1-19.

The Germinal Matrix

In the preterm infant, a highly vascular struc- ture known as the germinal matrix is found which is not seen in term infants or in adults. This tissue is a source of spongioblasts and neu- roblasts which migrate peripherally during the course of development to form adjacent struc- tures such as the cerebral cortex and basal gan- glia.[28–30] Histologic studies on injected fetal brains suggest the presence of an immature vas-

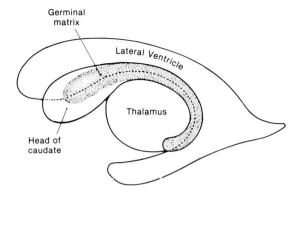

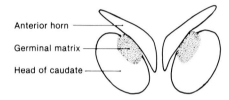

FIGURE 1-21. Relationship of the germinal matrix (*stippled area*) to adjacent lateral ventricle and developing caudate nucleus is illustrated as seen from side (*top*) and in coronal section (*bottom*).

cular rete within the germinal matrix that is gradually remodeled into the definitive capillary bed during the later stages of brain development.[28] The germinal matrix seems to be the source of the vast majority of intracranial hemorrhages in the preterm population.

This rudimentary embryonic structure is located inferolateral to the ependyma lining the floor of the lateral ventricle, and is also situated immediately superior to the developing head and body of the caudate nucleus (Fig. 1-21). This tissue is largest in the most premature infants and appears to involute during development, so that it is virtually absent by approximately 32 weeks of gestation.[28] Involution begins in the region of the body of the caudate nucleus and gradually proceeds anteriorly so that the subependymal tissue over the head of the caudate nucleus is the last region to involute. The clinical significance of the germinal matrix is discussed in subsequent chapters. The sonographic features of the region of the germinal matrix were discussed in Section 8.

Choroid Plexus

As has already been mentioned, the glomus of the choroid plexus in the atrium of the lateral ventricle should have a smooth contour in the normal infant, and any irregularity or "lumpiness" of the contour of the choroid should arouse suspicion of adjacent intraventricular hemorrhage. Not infrequently, however, the choroid plexus has an irregular contour, but no definite evidence of intraventricular hemorrhage or its sequelae is found in other images or in subsequent scans. Whether this indeed represents a variant of normal or a case of mild intraventricular hemorrhage that gradually resolves without sequelae has not been determined with certainty. In these situations, serial sonograms are most helpful to exclude treatable disease, that is, the development of hydrocephalus. More will be said in a subsequent chapter regarding the differentiation between the normal choroid plexus and small amounts of intraventricular hemorrhage.

Sylvian Fissure and Subarachnoid Spaces

The appearance of the Sylvian fissure varies with the gestational age of the infant.[24, 31] As pointed out by Jeanty et al., the frontal and temporal opercula that delineate the Sylvian fissure are not well formed in the preterm infant, so that the echo complex seen in this region in immature neonates actually represents the exposed surface of the insula.[31] The insular echo complex in the parasagittal view in the preterm infant often appears as a "flag" (Fig. 1-22). This may be contrasted with the appearance of the more gestationally mature Sylvian fissure shown in Fig. 1-18. One should not assume this continuous triangular echogenicity represents subarachnoid hemorrhage.

Laing and co-workers[32] demonstrated that all the subarachnoid spaces may be prominent in the fetus and the preterm neonate. Occasionally one may be able to define the surface of the brain or even separation of the apposing cerebral lobes in the area of the Sylvian or interhemispheric fissures (Fig. 1-23). Again, one must not mistake this normal variant for pathology.

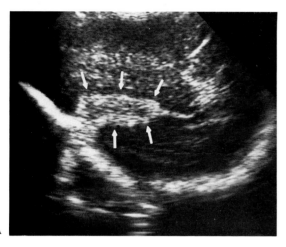

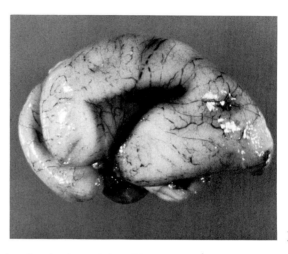

A

B

FIGURE 1-22. **A**, Angled parasagittal scan lateral to temporal horn of lateral ventricle in premature infant. Exposed surface of the insula appears as an echogenic flag-shaped area (*arrows*), contrasted by low-level echogenicity of frontal, temporal, and parietal opercula. **B**, Gross photograph of lateral surface of brain specimen in premature infant. Compare with Fig. 1-18.

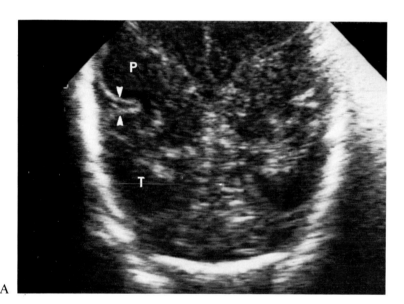

A

B

FIGURE 1-23. Normal subarachnoid space in preterm infant. Angled coronal section (**A**) shows separation of parietal (*P*) and temporal (*T*) lobes by a widened Sylvian fissure (*arrowheads*). Parasagittal section (**B**) shows surface of brain (*arrows*) to be separated from the skull by subarachnoid fluid.

FIGURE 1-24. Angled parasagittal scan through body and frontal and occipital horns of lateral ventricle. Note area of increased echogenicity (*arrows*) adjacent to trigone of the ventricle. This normal periventricular echogenicity is never as brightly echogenic as adjacent glomus of the choroid plexus (*open arrow*).

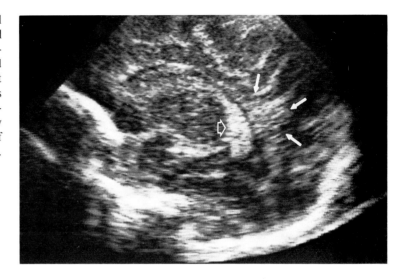

Periventricular Halo

Often an area of increased echogenicity can be identified about the lateral ventricles, particularly in the region of the trigone. This is most frequently encountered in the angled parasagittal images through the trigone of the lateral ventricle (Fig. 1-24), and is also seen on the high axial scans (Figs. 1-12 and 1-13). We have termed this the echogenic periventricular halo,[22] and it is seen to a variable degree in most normal scans. It is not certain whether this should be considered a normal variant or a scanning artifact; however, as no single normal structure seems to correspond to this area of echogenicity, it is probably best termed an artifact. The degree of echogenicity in this region is important: the normal halo is never as echogenic as the choroid plexus in the trigone. However, pathologic conditions demonstrating increased echogenicity in this area usually appear as bright as the adjacent choroid. If doubt exists, serial sonography or CT should be performed to establish the significance of the finding. If the periventricular echogenicity is pathologic, periventricular leukomalacia, later manifested as a conglomeration of tiny cystic spaces, is the almost universal sequela.

Summary

The normal anatomy of the neonatal brain as depicted with real-time ultrasound sector scanning has been presented along with similar sections of the neonatal brain for comparison. The brain of the newborn infant, particularly that of the preterm, differs substantially from the adult brain; these distinctions and certain commonly encountered variants from the norm have been illustrated and emphasized in the text. With an appreciation of the range of *normal,* the reader is invited to explore the various pathologic states as seen with real-time sonography in the following chapters.

References

1. Leksell L. Echoencephalography: detection of the intracranial complications following head injury. Acta Chir Scand 110:301–315, 1956.
2. Makow D, Real R. Emersion ultrasonic brain examination with 360-degree scan. Ultrasonics 3:75–80, 1965.
3. Garrett W, Kossoff G, Carpenter D, Radovanovich G. The octoson in use. In: Ultrasound in Medicine 2. White D, Barnes R, eds. Plenum, New York, 341–349, 1976.
4. Haber K, Wachter R, Christenson P, Vaucher Y, Sahn D, Smith J. Ultrasonic evaluation of intracranial pathology in infants: a new technique. Radiology 134:173–178, 1980.
5. Haber K. Automated water delay head scanning. In: Cranial Ultrasonography of Infants. Babcock D, Han B, eds. Williams and Wilkins, Baltimore, 105–139, 1981.
6. Ben-Ora A, Eddy L, Hatch G, Solida B. The anterior fontanelle as an acoustic window to the neonatal ventricular system. JCU 8:65–67, 1980.
7. London D, Carroll B, Enzmann D. Sonography of ventricular size and germinal matrix hemor-

rhage in premature infants. AJNR 1:295–300, 1980.

8. Grant E, Schellinger D, Borts F, McCullough D, Friedman G, Sivasubramanian K, Smith Y. Real-time sonography of the neonatal and infant head. AJNR 1:487–492, 1980.

9. Slovis T, Kuhns L. Real-time sonography of the brain through the anterior fontanelle. AJR 136:277–286, 1981.

10. Caffey J. Pediatric X-Ray Diagnosis, Vol. 1 (6th Ed.). Year Book, Chicago, 23, 1973.

11. Raimondi A. Pediatric Neuroradiology. Saunders, Philadelphia, 1972.

12. Smith W, Franklin T, Katakura K, Patrick J, Fry F, Eggleton R. A simple device to couple linear array transducers to neonatal heads for ultrasonic scanning of the brain. Radiology 137:838–839, 1980.

13. Mercker J, Blumhagen J, Brewer D. Echographic demonstration of extracerebral fluid collections with the lateral technique. J Ultrasound Med 2:265–269, 1983.

14. Pigadas A, Thompson J, Grube G. Normal infant brain anatomy: correlated real-time sonograms and brain specimens. AJNR 2:339–344, 1981.

15. Grant E, Schellinger D, Richardson J. Real-time ultrasonography of the posterior fossa. J Ultrasound Med 2:73–87, 1983.

16. Mack L, Alvord E. Neonatal cranial ultrasound: normal apperances. Semin Ultrasound 3:216–230, 1982.

17. Kossoff G, Garrett W, Radavanovich G. Ultrasonic atlas of normal brain of infant. Ultrasound Med Biol 1:259–266, 1974.

18. Johnson M, Rumack C. Ultrasonic evaluation of the neonatal brain. Radiol Clin North Am 18:117–131, 1980.

19. Shuman W, Rogers J, Mack L, Alvord E, Christie D. Real-time sonographic sector scanning of the neonatal cranium: technique and normal anatomy. AJNR 2:349–356, 1981.

20. Harwood-Nash D, Flodmark O. Diagnostic imaging of the neonatal brain: review and protocol. AJNR 3:103–115, 1982.

21. Horbar J, Leahy K, Lucey J. Ultrasound identification of lateral ventricular asymmetry in the human neonate. JCU 11:67–69, 1983.

22. Grant E, Schellinger D, Richardson J, Coffey M, Smirniotopoulous J. Echogenic periventricular halo: normal sonographic finding or neonatal cerebral hemorrhage. AJNR 4:43–46, 1983.

23. Bowie J, Kirks D, Rosenberg E, Clair M. Caudothalamic groove: value in identification of germinal matrix hemorrhage by sonography in preterm neonates. AJR 141:1317–1320, 1983.

24. Dorovini-Zis K, Dolman C. Gestational development of brain. Arch Pathol Lab Med 101:192–195, 1977.

25. Shaw C, Alvord E. Cava septi pellucidi et vergae: their normal and pathologic states. Brain 92:213–224, 1969.

26. Deck M. The lateral ventricles. In: Radiology of the skull and brain, Vol. 4, Newton T, Potts D, eds. Mosby, St. Louis, 1978.

27. Goodwin L, Quisling R. The neonatal cisterna magna: ultrasonic evaluation. Radiology 149: 691–695, 1983.

28. Pape K, Wigglesworth J. Hemorrhage, Ischemia and the Perinatal Brain. Lippincott, Philadelphia, 1979.

29. Hambleton G, Wigglesworth J. Origin of intraventricular hemorrhage in the preterm infant. Arch Dis Child 51:651–659, 1976.

30. Papile L, Burstein J, Bursten R, Koffler H. Incidence and evolution of subependymal and intraventricular hemorrhage: a study of infants with birth weights less than 1500 grams. J Pediatr 92:529–534, 1978.

31. Jeanty P, Chervenak F, Romero R, Michiels M, Hobbins J. The Sylvian fissure: a commonly mislabeled cranial landmark. J Ultrasound Med 3:15–18, 1984.

32. Laing F, Stamler C, Jeffrey B. Ultrasonography of the fetal subarachnoid space. J Ultrasound Med 2:29–32, 1983.

33. Key EAH, Retzius G. Studien in der Anatomie des Nervensystems und des Bindegewebes. Stockholm, Samson and Wallin, 1875.

2
Pathophysiology of Germinal Matrix-Related Hemorrhage and Ischemia

K.N. Siva Subramanian

Introduction

A wide variety of intracranial pathology is found in the newborn infant. Two unique lesions, however, affect the premature brain. On the basis of what is presently known, these two lesions superficially appear to have very different origins, yet both are rooted in the fetal anatomy and physiology that persist in the premature infant. The better known of these two lesions is germinal matrix-related hemorrhage (GMRH). Although four major forms of intracranial hemorrhage may affect newborn infants, only GMRH has been specifically related to gestational immaturity. The second lesion, periventricular leukomalacia (PVL), appears to be ischemic in nature and primarily affects the periventricular white matter. Although PVL is considerably less common than GMRH, it is acquiring increasing importance because it is almost invariably associated with poor developmental outcome, as will be seen in the chapter on follow-up of these infants.

Germinal Matrix-Related Hemorrhage

The site of origin of the vast majority of intracranial hemorrhages in preterm infants is in the germinal matrix.[1, 2] The germinal matrix zone is peculiar to the mammalian brain, and appears during embryonic development along the lateral ventricular margin.[3] This highly metabolically active structure consists of proliferating neuroectodermal cells and is richly vascularized. In comparison with the vessels supplying the relatively undifferentiated cerebral cortex, postmortem studies have shown that the vessels supplying the germinal matrix are very prominent between 24 and 32 weeks of gestation (Fig. 2-1). The size of Heubner's artery suggests that in fact a major portion of the entire blood supply of the fetal brain is directed toward this germinal matrix area (Fig. 2-2).[4]

Beyond 32 weeks gestational age, the neuroectodermal cells of the germinal matrix migrate toward the cerebral cortex with resultant disappearance of the matrix zone. Remodeling of the vascular bed also occurs around this time, and preferential flow is thereafter directed toward supplying the rapidly developing cortical mantle rather than the deeper structures that are so prominent during earlier gestational stages (Fig. 2-3). The blood vessels within the germinal matrix zone are extremely fragile; consisting of a single layer of endothelial cells, they can actually be considered capillaries.[5] In addition, these germinal matrix cells and vessels have little supporting stroma; they are therefore very vulnerable to damage and rupture when exposed to the stresses suffered by almost every preterm neonate during the perinatal period.

If the hemorrhage is severe enough, or if factors that would normally restrict the spread of hemorrhage are not present or are impaired, transependymal rupture of the initial germinal matrix hemorrhage may occur. In some instances, the hemorrhage may extend into the surrounding cerebral parenchyma. Once blood has found its way into the lateral ventricles in sufficient quantities, it may pass through the third and fourth ventricles and collect in the basilar cisterns of the brain, as illustrated by the

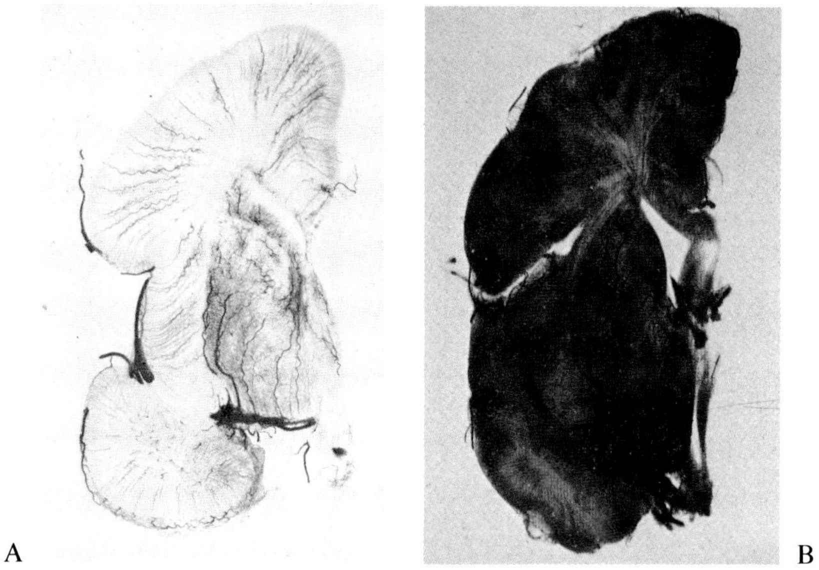

FIGURE 2-1. Postmortem studies of the brain at 24 (**A**) and 34 (**B**) weeks of gestational age. From Pape and Wigglesworth.[4]

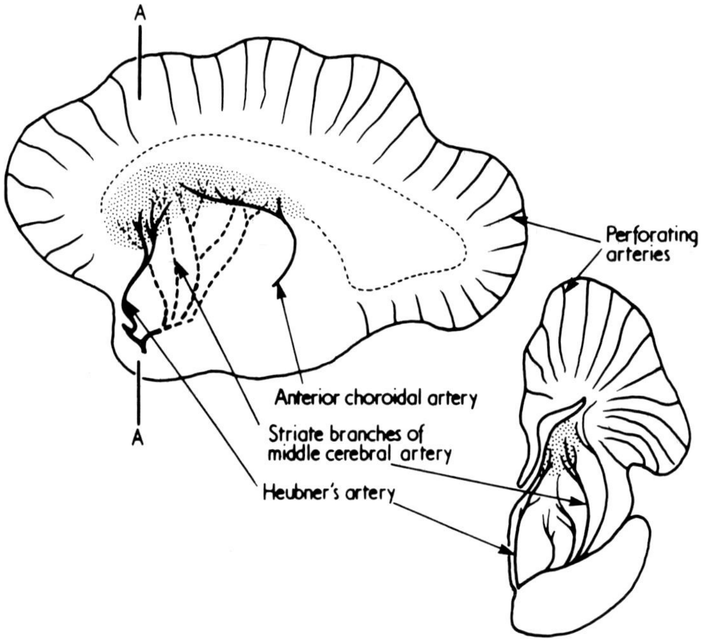

FIGURE 2-2. Arterial supply at 29 weeks gestation. From Hambleton and Wigglesworth.[2]

FIGURE 2-3. Changes in arterial pattern of cerebrum between 24 and 34 weeks gestation. From Wigglesworth and Pape.[20]

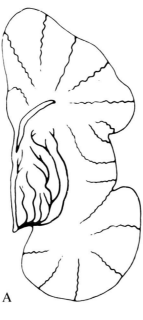

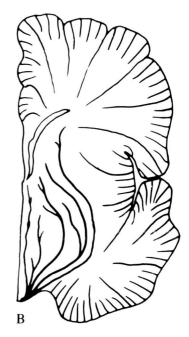

A

24 weeks

B

34 weeks

pathologic specimen in Fig. 3-6 C. In addition to actually blocking the normal egress of cerebrospinal fluid (CSF) at certain narrow points in the ventricular system, blood in the subarachnoid cisterns may cause an obliterative arachnoiditis that results in the disruption of normal CSF flow dynamics and eventually leads to nonobstructive hydrocephalus. In addition, parenchymal hemorrhage appears to lead to direct destruction of brain substance, and in every instance a porencephalic cyst replaces the original hematoma.[6]

Ischemic Lesions/Periventricular Leukomalacia

Infarction of both grey and white matter during the perinatal period is of major importance as an etiologic factor in mental retardation and specific neurologic deficits.[7] The site of ischemic damage varies, depending on gestational maturity. In term infants, anoxic damage primarily affects the grey matter and the basal ganglia, frequently resulting in global loss of brain tissue or cerebral atrophy. In premature

infants, ischemic necrosis mainly affects the periventricular white matter, causing what is termed periventricular leukomalacia (PVL).

PVL is the direct result of infarction in arterial boundary zones, or as they are frequently called elsewhere in the body, watershed circulatory regions. These are areas that are particularly vulnerable to infarction, because they lie at the edges of two major arterial circulatory systems and are therefore not well supplied with blood nutrients by either artery. In term infants and in adults, the arterial boundary zones are located between the three major cerebral arteries, leaving the cerebral cortex and adjacent subcortical white matter most vulnerable. In the premature infant, however, the watershed zones are located in the periventricular white matter adjacent to the external margins of the lateral ventricles. These zones are situated approximately 3–10 mm from the ventricular wall. They lie between the terminal distributions of penetrating ventriculofugal arteries, which course from the choroid plexus peripherally, and the branches of the ventriculopetal parenchymal arteries originating at the surface of the brain (Fig. 2-4). The ventriculofu-

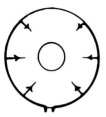

A. Ventriculopetal

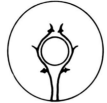

B. Ventriculofugal

FIGURE 2-4. Arterial pattern of the brain. From Wigglesworth and Pape.[20]

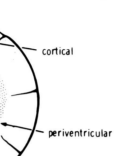

cortical

periventricular

C. Boundary Zones

gal vessels increase in number with increasing gestational age; the relative paucity in the premature infant targets the periventricular white matter as the structure most prone to ischemic infarction. Although studies directed toward the understanding of the basis of GMRH have been relatively few, studies directed toward an understanding of the factors involved with periventricular infarction are practically nonexistent. One may postulate that, in contrast to GMRH, decreases in cerebral perfusion may result in infarction.

Periventricular infarction affects the regions about the corona radiata and the centrum semiovale anteriorly, and the internal and external sagittal striations above the trigones of the lateral ventricles in the parietooccipital area.[8] This anatomic distribution places the internal and external capsules, the motor cortex, and the visual and speech centers at greatest risk for damage. The corticospinal tracts descending to the legs are the most vulnerable, because they lie closest to the ventricular margins (Fig. 2-5). The clinical sequelae of PVL were, in fact, very accurately described by W.J. Little[9] in 1843; " . . . mental retardation and spasticity of all the limbs . . . the spasticity was not al-

ways symmetrical, and the legs were more severely afflicted than the arms. . . .".

The neuropathologic characteristics of PVL were also initially described more than a century ago in separate papers published by Virchow[10] and Hayem[11] in the 1860s. In the next decade, Parrot[12] more completely delineated the "infarction, hemorrhage and diffuse interstitial steatosis in the deep white matter" and attributed the lesion to a "nutritional and circulatory disturbance occuring in an actively developing brain." He stressed the high association with prematurity, an observation originally made by Little in 1843 in his "Course of Lectures on the Deformities of the Human Frame."

It was Banker and Larroche,[13] however, who in 1962 presented the classic detailed description of the sequential pathologic changes of PVL, starting with the pathognomonic "coagulation necrosis" of the periventricular white matter through the stages of microglial, astrocytic, and vascular proliferation, and followed eventually by ependymal loss. Thus a series of histologic changes ranging from coagulation necrosis to axonal disintegration, reactive astrocytosis, and finally liquefication and cavitation occurs in PVL.

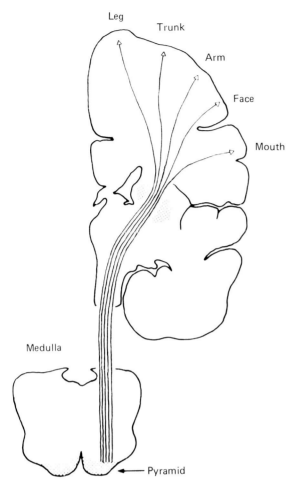

Leg

Trunk

Arm

Face

Mouth

Medulla

Pyramid

FIGURE 2-5. Relationship of periventricular necrosis to corticospinal from tracts. Pape and Wigglesworth.[4]

Physiology of Cerebral Circulation

The effect of various physiologic factors on the cerebral circulation of the adult is well known, but data on the developing fetus and premature neonate are very limited. Animal and adult human studies have suggested that changes in arterial blood pressure within a specific range have no direct effect on cerebral blood flow (CBF). This autoregulatory effect, however, may be lost if blood pressure falls too low or rises too high. Other factors, including changes in arterial oxygen, carbon dioxide, and pH levels, and various drugs such as aminophylline and morphine, have also been shown to affect CBF in adults. Studies in fetal lambs show that CBF is markedly influenced by changes in systemic blood pressure and the other factors just described.[14] These same studies also suggested that CBF probably increases with increasing maturity in utero. Although many of the adult cerebral circulatory responses are present at birth, Reivich and Myers[15] showed that this control is easily impaired by birth asphyxia in term monkeys. Whether animal and adult human data can be extrapolated to preterm infants is, of course, unknown; but many of these mechanisms seem to be operative in infants. Lou et al.[16] studied a group of premature infants with Xenon clearance technique soon after birth. They concluded that the rate of CBF in the premature infant is lower than in the adult, and the relationship between CBF and systolic blood pressure is linear. The apparent CBF increases immediately after birth nearly twofold and then after three hours is relatively stable.[17] Thus, autoregulation in premature infants seems to be very labile and pressure-passive. Separate studies by different methods in premature infants with respiratory distress syndrome and/or asphyxia demonstrated that infants are not capable of autoregulation of CBF, which varied from 17–55 ml/100 g/min at 3–12 hr of age.[16,18]

Pathogenesis of GMRH/PVL

Beyond the physiologic factors outlined above, other authors have suspected that mechanical factors may play a part in the origin of GMRH. These factors include compression, stasis, or frank mechanical tearing of the fragile capillaries.[19,20] Other disease processes such as disseminated intravascular coagulation (DIC), hypernatremia, or excessive fibrinolytic activity in the germinal matrix may play some role in either the initial hemorrhagic event or its further spread. Marked increases in CBF occur in many clinical situations, such as apnea,[17] pneumothorax[21], and other air-leak syndromes.[22] Suctioning[23] and rapid volume expansion[24] may also lead to GMRH. Overall, it is generally accepted that significant increases in CBF in association with the fragile vessels in the germinal matrix lead to most intracranial hemorrhages in the preterm neonate. In addi-

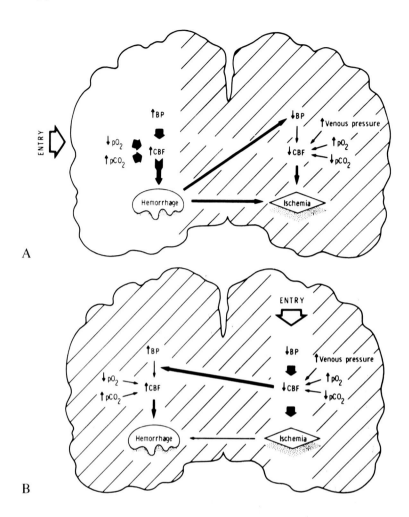

FIGURE 2-6. Classic two-part model of hemorrhage and ischemia. *BP* = blood pressure; *CBF* = cerebral blood flow. From Wigglesworth and Pape.[25]

A

B

tion, multifactorial mechanisms such as those just discussed may actually coexist in causing germinal matrix hemorrhage.

The factors that set the stage for GMRH/PVL in premature infants include prematurity, the presence of a highly metabolically active and fragile subependymal matrix, increased blood supply to this area, impaired or poorly developed autoregulation, increased cerebral venous pressure, endothelial damage, and periventricular fibrinolytic activity as described earlier. The classic two-part scheme (Fig. 2-6) for the origins of GMRH and PVL was espoused by Wigglesworth and Pape.[25] Our diagram has been modified to reflect the factors that set the stage for both hemorrhagic and ischemic lesions in the preterm neonate (Fig. 2-7). In this model, hypoxemia and hypercarbia, either alone or in combination, result in vascu-

lar dilatation. Any increase in systemic blood pressure coupled with vasodilatation leads to a marked increase in CBF. This is particularly pertinent in the preterm infant because of impaired or immature cerebral autoregulatory capacity. These factors, as shown in our model, set the stage for capillary rupture in the germinal matrix. If the hemorrhage is not contained as a result of increased fibrinolytic activity, DIC, and/or lack of supporting stroma in the germinal matrix, blood may rupture into the ventricle or invade the surrounding parenchyma. The hemorrhage itself may then lead to ischemia due to reactive vasospasm and pressure effect. Further compounding the situation is the possible fall of blood pressure, resulting from the loss of large quantities of blood into the ventricles or the surrounding cerebral parenchyma.

FIGURE 2-7. Modified model for both hemorrhage and ischemic lesions in the preterm infant.

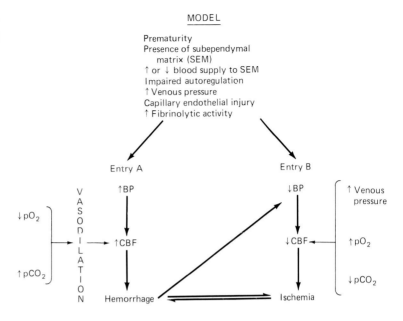

The opposite scenario may also be worked through this model, when the infant is subjected to hypotension. Hypotension may occur for various reasons; asphyxia and sepsis are among the most common offenders in the premature age group. CBF decreases in these premature infants who are subjected to hypotension, and the persistent hypotension can lead to ischemia. Such ischemia can result in capillary endothelial injury. Further, in asphyxia and sepsis, hypoxic or endotoxic capillary endothelial damage occurs frequently. Attempts by the physician at this time to improve the overall condition of the infant by correcting acidosis, hypoxia, and/or hypercarbia may actually then lead to cerebral hyperperfusion, which may then result in rupture of the damaged capillaries causing GMRH.

The exact reasons for the frequency of both hemorrhagic and ischemic lesions in the preterm brain are at best poorly understood. The importance of PVL is only beginning to become evident, and although GMRH has been studied for many years, much work remains in the future. Further research into the causes of GMRH and ischemia is obviously needed. Such investigations have been particularly difficult because of a lack of an appropriate animal model even though sheep and beagle puppies have been used with moderate success. Careful evaluation of newer imaging techniques, such as magnetic resonance imaging (MRI) and positron emission tomography (PET), may better define the extent of cerebral injury, especially that of ischemia. Newer areas of research include the evaluation of brain temperature and changes in sleep states and we hope the future will yield a better understanding of this complex pathology. As will be seen in the following chapters, the imaging and even the follow-up of these lesions assumes greater clarity with an understanding of the underlying anatomy, pathology, and physiology.

References

1. Leech RW, Kohnen P. Subependymal and intraventricular hemorrhages in the newborn. Am J Pathol 77:465–475, 1974.
2. Hambleton G, Wigglesworth JS. Origin of intraventricular hemorrhage in the preterm infant. Arch Dis Child 51:651–659, 1976.
3. Rorke LB. Hemorrhages. In: Pathology of Perinatal Brain Injury. Rorke LB, ed. Raven, New York, 15, 1982.
4. Pape KE, Wigglesworth JS. Hemorrhage, ischemia and the perinatal brain. Clinics in Developmental Medicine, NOS 69/70. William Heineman, London, 1979.
5. Rorke LB. Hemorrhages. In: Pathology of Perinatal Brain Injury. Rorke LB, ed. Raven, New York, 15, 1982.

6. Schellinger D, Grant EG, Richardson JD. Cystic PVL sonographic and CT findings. AJNR 5:439–445, 1984.

7. De Rueck J, Chattha AS, Richardson EP Jr. Pathogenesis and evolution of PVL in infancy. Arch Neurol 27:229–236, 1972.

8. Leech RW, Alvard EC Jr. Morphological variations in PVL. Am J Pathol 74:591–602, 1974.

9. Little WJ. Course of lectures on the deformities of the human frame. Lecture VIII. Lancet I:318–322, 1843.

10. Virchow R. Ueber interstitielle Encephalitis. Virchow's Arch [Path Anat] 44:472–476, 1868.

11. Hayem G. Etudes sur les diverses formes d'encephalitis. Thesis, Doctorate in Medicine, Paris. 1868.

12. Parrot MD. Étude sur le ramollissement de l'encéphale chez le nouveau-né. Arch Physiol Nouv Pathol (Paris) 5:59–73, (1873).

13. Banker BQ, Larroche JC. Periventricular leukomalacia of infancy: A form of neonatal anoxic encephalopathy. Arch Neurol 7:386–410, 1962.

14. Rudolph AM, Heymann MA. Circulating changes during growth in the fetal lamb. Cir Res 26:289–299, 1970.

15. Reivich M, Myers RE. Regional cerebral blood flow during prolonged partial asphyxia. Research in Cerebral Circulation. Meyer JS, Reivich M, Lechner H, Eichorn O, eds. 5th International Salzburg Conference. Thomas, Springfield, 216–227, 1972.

16. Lou HC, Lassen NA, Friis-Hansen B. Low cerebral blood flow in hypotensive perinatal distress. Acta Neurol 56:343–352, 1977.

17. Cooke RWI, Rolfe P, Howat P. Apparent cerebral blood-flow in newborns with respiratory distress. Dev Med Child Neurol 21:154–160, 1979.

18. Cooke RWI, Rolfe P, Howat P. A technique for the non-invasive estimation of cerebral blood flow in the newborn infant. J Med Eng Technol 1:263–266, 1977.

19. Newton TH, Gooding CA. Compression of superior sagittal sinus by neonatal calvarial molding. Radiology 115:635–639, 1975.

20. Kosmetatos N, Williams ML. Effect of positioning and head banding on intracranial pressure in the premature infant. Pediatr Res 12:553, 1978.

21. Hill A, Perlman JM, Volpe JJ. Relationship of pneumothorax to occurrence of intraventricular hemorrhage in the premature newborn. Pediatrics 69:144–149, 1982.

22. Dykes FD, Lazzara A, Ahmann P, Blumenstein B, Schwartz J, Brann AW. Intraventricular hemorrhage: A prospective evaluation of etiopathogenesis. Pediatrics 66:42–49, 1980.

23. Perlman JM, Volpe JJ. Suctioning in the preterm infant: Effects on cerebral blood flow velocity, intracranial pressure and arterial blood pressure. Pediatrics 72:329–334, 1983.

24. Goddard-Finegold J, Armstrong D, Zeller RS. Intraventricular hemorrhage following volume expansion after hypovolemic hypotension in the newborn beagle. J Pediatr 100:796–799, 1982.

25. Wigglesworth JS, Pape KE. An integrated model for hemorrhage and ischemic lesions in the newborn brain. Early Hum Dev 2:179–199, 1978.

3
Neurosonography: Germinal Matrix-Related Hemorrhage

Edward G. Grant

Introduction

The radiologist has long been essential in the diagnosis of diseases that affect the premature neonate. The chest radiograph is necessary to establish the presence and severity of hyaline membrane disease and to differentiate it from other diseases that affect premature lungs. Similarly, the abdominal film is essential in monitoring the neonatal bowel. Only recently, however, has significant attention been directed toward imaging of the brain, as a greater percentage of premature neonates have begun to survive beyond the immediate perinatal period. In the very young, the central nervous system (CNS) can easily be overlooked. With the exception of a relatively small minority of neonates with massive intracranial hemorrhage, pathology in the premature CNS does not cause immediate death. Devastating intracranial pathology is, in fact, most frequently asymptomatic. Only after premature neonates were routinely evaluated using the computed tomography (CT) scanner did the frequency of intracranial pathology in the preterm neonate actually become apparent.[1] The anatomy and pathophysiology that underlie these processes have already been discussed in prior chapters, and we shall now take a detailed look at their sonographic features.

Before proceeding, however, certain guidelines must be laid down in an effort to decide which patients are to be scanned and when, since we are dealing with a largely asymptomatic population. To decide who shall be scanned, we require a strict definition of prematurity. Simply defined, neonates with a germinal ma-

trix and an immature vascular circulation are neurologically premature; infants with a more mature circulation and without a germinal matrix are not. Intracranial hemorrhage and infarction are quite unusual in the term infant, and differ greatly in their etiology and sonographic features from hemorrhage or infarction encountered in the preterm neonate.[2-6] We shall consider neonates of 32 weeks or less gestational age premature; after this time, the cerebral circulation more closely resembles that which is seen in term infants, and the germinal matrix usually is completely involuted. One rarely finds significant cerebroventricular hemorrhage (CVH) in neonates who are more than 32 weeks gestational age.[7-11] A specific demarcation between term and premature is of great importance; all premature neonates should undergo at least two cranial sonograms. Such routine and intensive scanning is costly and time consuming, and is not warranted for neonates who are not at a high risk for intracranial pathology.

Many authors have used birthweight as the determining factor in their scanning routines[12-14]; we feel this is not optimal. Although the overall percentage of neonates with intracranial pathology increases as birthweight decreases, it has been our experience that "small-for-gestational-age" neonates have a low frequency of intracranial pathology. This reflects their gestationally mature CNS, and suggests that it is the state of CNS maturity and not birthweight that determines the risk for intracranial pathology in most neonates.

Although routine cranial sonography is necessary for all neonates of 32 weeks gestational age or less, neonates between 33 and 36 weeks should be scanned in certain clinical situations. A good example is an infant with severe pulmonary disease but of 34 weeks gestational age. First, the gestational age may have been incorrectly estimated either by in utero parameters[15, 16] or by the routine postnatal evaluations such as the widely used "Dubowitz" scale.[17] Second, the child with respiratory disease will experience many of the stresses of a more premature neonate: Even if the germinal matrix is absent, this baby is undoubtedly at a higher risk for intracranial pathology than the normal term neonate without such stress. Liberal use of intracranial sonography is therefore urged in this borderline mature group, especially in those neonates subjected to severe stress or hypoxia.

The premise that all neonates of 32 weeks or less gestational age require cranial sonograms deserves detailed examination. Prior to the landmark article of Burstein et al. in 1979,[1] it was held by some that CVH was a preterminal event.[18] Many autopsy series reported a high incidence of CVH[10, 19], but its occurrence in the living neonate was felt to be unusual. The classic clinical picture of the child with CVH was generally thought to consist of hypotension, decreased hematocrit, severe apnea and bradycardia, and seizure activity.[20, 21] This "catastrophic event" is not commonly encountered, and the 1979 study proved it was the exception and not the rule. This study of cranial CT scans performed on 100 consecutive premature neonates, regardless of symptoms, showed 43% to have some form of CVH.

Other investigators have found even higher percentages of intracranial hemorrhage in their population.[13, 22–25] It became apparent that, although some neonates do manifest the clinical signs of CVH, most do not. Clinically, there is no simple way to differentiate the majority of neonates with sometimes severe CVH from those without it. Posthemorrhagic hydrocephalus (PHH) and porencephaly may also go unnoticed clinically until, in the case of hydrocephalus, it becomes severe.[21, 26–28] Periventricular leukomalacia (PVL) actually seems to manifest no immediate clinical abnormalities, and it can only be diagnosed in its early stages by radiologic means. One must, therefore, scan all prematures to diagnose and follow these common but silent cerebral insults.

There are many specific reasons for performing cranial sonography. First, a direct relationship has been demonstrated between the maximum amount of intraventricular hemorrhage (IVH) and the severity of PHH that will develop later.[28–36] Early cranial sonography can identify which neonates are at risk for significant PHH in the first week or so of life. Those with significant intraventricular hematoma demand close follow-up for ventricular enlargement. A second important reason for routine sonographic evaluation of the preterm brain is the identification of intraparenchymal cerebral insults. All series thus far show that children with intraparenchymal hemorrhage invariably develop porencephalic cysts.[37–40] Additionally, those with PVL must be identified. Clinical and autopsy studies suggest a poor outcome in many neonates with large parenchymal hemorrhages[31, 41, 42] or PVL.[43–45] Therefore, early sonographic observations may have far-reaching prognostic implications that may aid clinicians in forming an overall picture of a particular infant.

Cranial sonography may also help to explain an acute clinical deterioration: Was intracranial pathology the cause? The positive sonogram may, however, be misleading. If a large intracranial hemorrhage is held responsible for clinical deterioration, the real culprit, which may require immediate treatment, may be overlooked. On the other hand, the existence of severe intracranial pathology in conjunction with multisystem failure may lead the neonatalogist to a different approach to such a child. The early sonographic diagnosis of intracranial pathology is therefore of great importance both in establishing a possible cause for a clinical deterioration and as part of establishing the overall clinical picture of a particular neonate.

In addition to the original diagnostic ultrasound to establish the presence and severity of CVH and/or PVL, follow-up scans are also important. These follow-up scans are imperative in neonates with intraventricular hemorrhages because they are at high risk for PHH. Selected neonates with PVL require significant follow-up as well. Although the parenchymal insult is neither treatable nor apt to require follow-up, simultaneous IVH is not uncommon in these infants. Children with a combination of PVL and

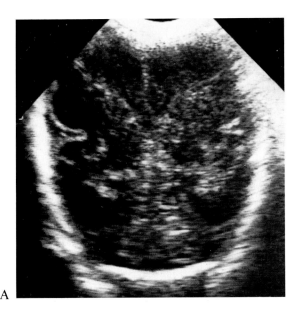

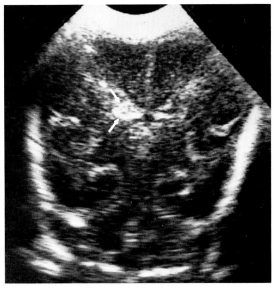

FIGURE 3-1. Serial angled coronal sections from 26-week gestational age neonate at 1, 2, and 3 days of age. Scan on day 1 (**A**) is normal. Scan on day 2 (**B**) shows interval development of large germinal matrix hemorrhage (GMH) (*arrows*). Severe apnea, bradycardia, and hypotension occurred between days 2 and 3; hematocrit fell precipitously. Final scan on day 3 (**C**) shows progression of hemorrhage; note large intraventricular/intraparenchymal hematoma on right (*arrowheads*) and intraventricular hematoma (IVH) on left (*curved arrow*). Child died on day 4.

IVH often have protracted and very difficult clinical courses and may require continued cranial sonography throughout their hospital course and beyond.[46]

Partridge et al.[47] have attempted to identify the optimal times for routine scanning by evaluating diagnostic yield. We feel that their method offers an excellent initial scanning routine which allows little room for pathology to go unnoticed but does not demand an excessive number of sonograms. The first routine scan should be performed between 4 and 7 days of age. By

that time the vast majority of CVHs will have taken place.[12, 47] Additionally, since germinal matrix-related hemorrhage is not an all-at-once phenomenon,[48] progression to more severe involvement may occur over a matter of days but will undoubtedly maximize before 1 week (Fig. 3-1, A–C).

A second sonogram at 2 weeks of age should also be performed routinely. By this time, those children developing significant hydrocephalus can be identified. Any unusual late CVH that has occurred between 7 and 14 days of life should also be apparent. In our nursery, if a child has two routine sonograms that are normal, further scanning is not done. If abnormal, weekly sonograms are needed to establish a trend with regard to ventricular size. Since enlargement, stabilization, and, finally, decrease in ventricular size seem to be the natural history of most cases of PHH, weekly follow-up is essential until stabilization of ventricular size is identified. Once stabilization, and, more importantly, decreasing ventricular size are noted, one may scan at 2- to 3- (or more) week intervals or until the ventricles return to normal or near-normal size. In children in whom continued ventricular enlargement is the trend, therapy in the form of serial lumbar punctures or shunting may be required. After institution of therapy, these children must continue with weekly scans until a trend toward decreasing ventricular size is established. Much more will be said regarding PHH and its follow-up in the section on IVH.

A brief note should also be included about nonroutine scanning before 7 days of age and routine scanning before discharge from the hospital. For children with especially difficult clinical courses, the clinician may be aided in his or her decision process by early knowledge of the status of the brain. A sonogram prior to 7 days of life may therefore be advisable. Finally, a predischarge sonogram is urged for all infants. We have occasionally seen a patient with unexplained ventriculomegaly at discharge, although cause was apparent on early routine scans. Cerebral atrophy is best diagnosed on late ultrasound examinations, and PVL may not be obvious in its early phase; the characteristic periventricular cysts may not appear until 20 or more days of age.[49] Because the prognosis in children with atrophy and/or PVL is so poor, one must be especially careful that they are never overlooked.

In summary, all neonates of 32 weeks gestational age or less require routine cranial sonography. The optimal timing for the initial sonogram is at 1 week of age, and a second scan should be performed at 2 weeks. If both are normal, further scanning is not necessary. Continued weekly scans are essential in all infants with developing PHH until stabilization of ventricular size is achieved either with or without therapy. In general, with stabilization of ven-

tricular size one may decrease the scanning interval to 2 or 3 weeks. Because certain forms of pathology may not manifest themselves early on, a routine predischarge sonogram is also urged.

The Diagnosis of Germinal Matrix-Related Hemorrhage

Germinal matrix-related hemorrhage (GMRH) is the most common cerebral insult that affects the premature infant. Although the occurrence of intracranial hemorrhage in association with prematurity was long known to the neuropathologist, it could not be confidently diagnosed premortem before the advent of the CT scanner. CT scanning is a highly accurate method of diagnosing and characterizing GMRH; however, a number of inherent properties of the technology, foremost among which being its lack of portability, preclude its use as a screening procedure. Although infant neuroimaging with ultrasound had been elegantly accomplished in 1975 by Garrett and co-workers,[50] little attention was given to its possibilities until 1980, when a number of published reports[51–53] indicated that portable, real-time ultrasound could quite successfully image GMRH and its complications. Although earlier reports of the success of both conventional static ultrasound[54–56] and waterpath[57] scanning were promising, it was the portability of the sector scanner that had the greatest impact.

Almost immediately after the discovery that ultrasound could accurately diagnose CVH came investigation into which early sonographic abnormalities could serve as prognostic indicators. Follow-up studies show that, indeed, sonographic characterization of early hemorrhage does allow one to statistically predict the outcome. Most authors used the maximum severity or extent of the hemorrhage as their major diagnostic variable. We shall use a system adapted from the sonographic studies of Fleischer et al.[29, 58] and Shankaran.[31] Fleischer's work demonstrated that the size and extent of the original hemorrhage correlates directly with the severity of later sonographic abnormalities such as PHH and porencephaly. Other authors have closely corroborated this.[31–36] Shankarhan's study, on the other hand, indicated that actual clinical outcome also closely parallels early sonographic abnormalities. Because both sonographic and clinical prognoses are so directly dependent on the nature of the original hemorrhagic event, the characterization and classification of GMRH assumes a very important role for both the medical neuroimager and the neonatologist.

For the purpose of clarity, we shall use a simple classification system based on the maximum severity of the hemorrhage. Along the lines proposed by most authors, the grades of hemorrhage shall be I through IV. Increasing grades of hemorrhages correspond to increasing severity. Grade I CVH is confined to one or both germinal matrices. In Grade II CVH, the germinal matrix hemorrhage has ruptured into the ventricular system, but is not of sufficient size or pressure to significantly expand the ventricle with hematoma. Grade III CVH is similar to Grade II but of sufficient magnitude to expand the ventricles with blood. Obviously, Grades II and III are both properly termed IVH, and the actual distinction is somewhat arbitrary, since IVH of moderate proportions is occasionally encountered. The distinction is, however, more than semantic; the prognosis of children with IVH is influenced considerably by the size of the original hematoma. In the literature, authors have sometimes been vague on this subject. Because we have found such a difference in prognoses when comparing children with small versus large IVHs, I would like to reemphasize that our classification system is based entirely on the size of the hemorrhage and has nothing whatsoever to do with the ventriculomegaly that so frequently follows IVH. PHH is a sequel; hydrocephalus does not change the original grade, although the two are closely related. The onset of ventriculomegaly following a small (Grade II) hemorrhage does not imply *any* progression of the original event, merely a secondary complication.

Although the distinction between Grades II and III may be somewhat controversial, Grade IV CVH has almost always been straightforward. This most severe form of GMRH signifies that the original bleeding has spread not only into the ventricles but into the parenchyma as well. Not only would most authors concur about the diagnosis of Grade IV CVH, but most would also agree it has the worst prognosis. The

major question that seems at present to surround the diagnosis of Grade IV or intraparenchymal hemorrhage is its relationship and differentiation from PVL. At times this may be difficult, if not impossible, and it is my belief that the entire concept of intraparenchymal insults needs to be reexamined. We shall approach the concept of Grade IV hemorrhage from the classical standpoint and consider it an extension of a germinal matrix hemorrhage.

Each of the three major forms of GMRH (germinal matrix-related, intraventricular, and intraparenchymal hemorrhage) will be discussed separately, although in large hemorrhages all three coexist. This will considerably simplify the discussion because not only does each of the major forms of CVH have specific sonographic characteristics, each has specific sequelae. The use of this simple classification system should enable the neurosonographer not only to anticipate the severity and likelihood of short-term complication such as PHH and porencephaly, but to also define the statistical possibilities for the future of a given neonate as far as follow-up presently permits.

Grade I: Germinal Matrix Hemorrhage

Germinal matrix hemorrhage (GMH) is also known as subependymal or germinal layer hemorrhage. It is considered the most benign form of CVH. No studies thus far have shown any abnormality in association with isolated GMH.[31, 41, 42, 45] Occurring alone, it almost represents an incidental finding. The importance of hemorrhage into this fetal structure lies in its all-too-frequent extension into the adjacent ventricle or cerebral parenchyma. In this case, the "incidental" GMH may have a devastating effect on large portions of the brain. Alone, GMH should never be associated with PHH. In the occasional neonate diagnosed as having isolated GMH and associated ventricular enlargement, one must question the possibility of a small amount of IVH that was unnoticed by routine scanning. Since isolated GMH is entirely extraventricular, if cases of atrophy are excluded, there is no reason for subsequent ventriculomegaly.

The typical sonographic appearance of GMH is an echogenic focus at or directly anterior to the caudothalamic notch.[59] On parasagittal sec-

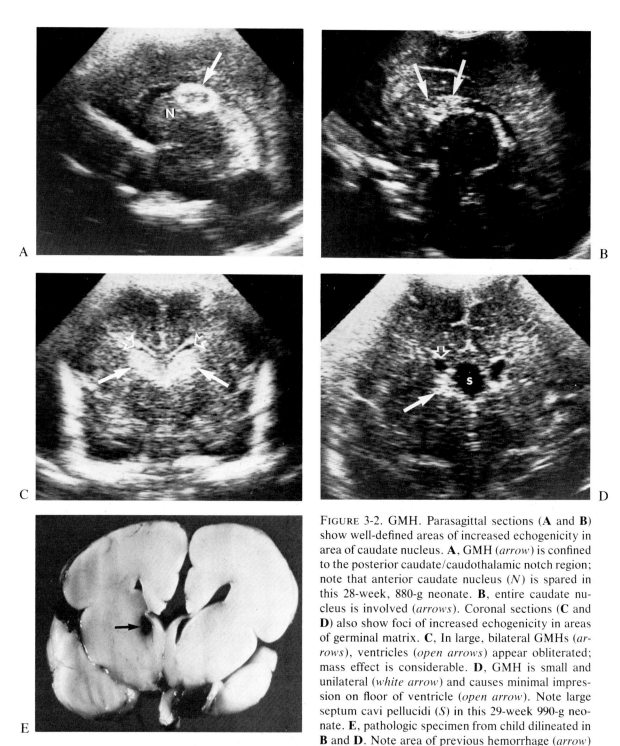

FIGURE 3-2. GMH. Parasagittal sections (**A** and **B**) show well-defined areas of increased echogenicity in area of caudate nucleus. **A**, GMH (*arrow*) is confined to the posterior caudate/caudothalamic notch region; note that anterior caudate nucleus (*N*) is spared in this 28-week, 880-g neonate. **B**, entire caudate nucleus is involved (*arrows*). Coronal sections (**C** and **D**) also show foci of increased echogenicity in areas of germinal matrix. **C**, In large, bilateral GMHs (*arrows*), ventricles (*open arrows*) appear obliterated; mass effect is considerable. **D**, GMH is small and unilateral (*white arrow*) and causes minimal impression on floor of ventricle (*open arrow*). Note large septum cavi pellucidi (*S*) in this 29-week 990-g neonate. **E**, pathologic specimen from child dilineated in **B** and **D**. Note area of previous hemorrhage (*arrow*) on right.

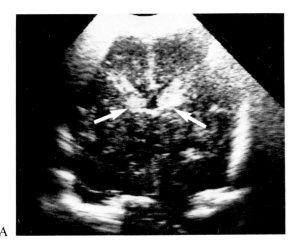

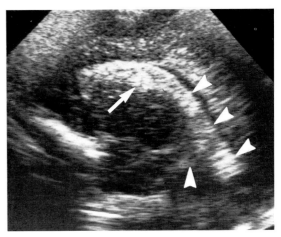

A

B

FIGURE 3-3. Large bilateral GMHs (*arrows*). **A**, Coronal section. **B**, Parasagittal orientation shows true extent of hemorrhage. Beyond germinal matrix component, entire posterior ventricle is filled with hematoma (*arrowheads*); therefore, this is a Grade III IVH.

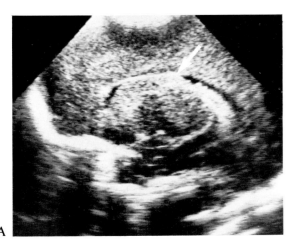

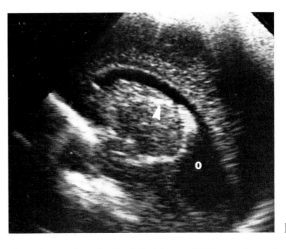

A

B

FIGURE 3-4. Maturation of GMH. Original scan at 3 days (**A**) shows typical echogenic GMH (*arrow*). Predischarge sonogram at 6 weeks (**B**) shows residual linear echogenicity in area beneath caudate nucleus (*arrowhead*). Occipital horn (*O*) has enlarged somewhat since earlier scan; a small amount of intraventricular hematoma was noted on intervening study.

tions, increased echogenicity may be localized to the area of the caudothalamic notch or posterior caudate nucleus or may extend some distance anteriorly, sometimes involving the entire caudate nucleus. In the coronal orientation, an echogenic focus is identified in a corresponding location that often impresses on the inferolateral border of the ventricular body (Fig. 3-2, A–D). GMH may be unilateral or bilateral, and the echogenicity may persist for some time, up to 2 months in some cases. At times the subependymal hemorrhage may be so extensive that the ventricular lumen will be obliterated, making differentiation between GMH and true IVH impossible on coronal sections alone (Fig. 3-3, A and B). Hambleton and Wigglesworth described a varying location for GMH depending on gestational age: anterior caudate nucleus at 24–26 weeks, middle at 26–28 weeks, and the area of the caudothalamic notch subse-

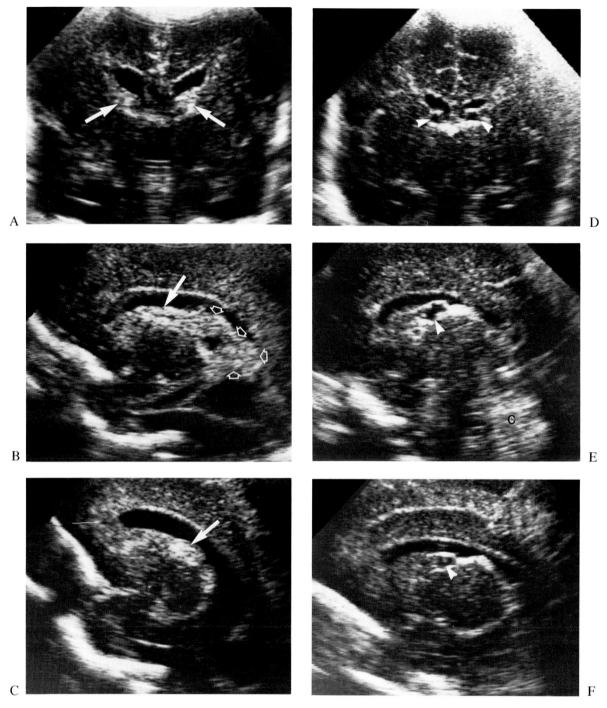

FIGURE 3-5. Maturation of GMH. Coronal (**A**), and right (**B**) and left (**C**) parasagittal sections show large bilateral GMHs (*arrows*). Note moderate ventriculomegaly and large right IVH (*open arrows*) at 1 week. Corresponding sonographic sections at 8 weeks (**D**–**F**) show formation of bilateral subependymal cysts (*arrowheads*). Such subependymal cysts frequently appear almost in the midline on parasagittal sections. Note cerebellar vermis (*C*) in same section as subependymal cyst in **E**.

quently.[60] The germinal matrix extends far posteriorly in very premature neonates; theoretically, therefore, GMH could originate in almost any portion of the ventricular floor.[10] Figure 3-1, however, clearly illustrates that these hemorrhages may vary, although the examples given do not correspond to the expected locations according to the gestational ages.

The original echogenic germinal matrix hematoma eventually matures. It may disappear entirely, or a thin echogenic line may remain that may represent an area of scarring or fibrosis (Fig. 3-4, A and B). The most curious situation, however, is the evolution of the hematoma into a subependymal cyst (Fig. 3-5, A–F). The significance of these cysts is uncertain, and no one has yet followed them closely over time either sonographically or clinically. We have recently examined one neonate in whom a subependymal cyst had resolved on a follow-up scan obtained at 10 months of age. Larroche described the pathology of these cysts in 1972.[61, 62] Similar subependymal cysts have also been identified by Shackelford et al. in term neonates without GMH, but the etiology in this group is somewhat more obscure. Their series most commonly associated nonhemorrhagic subependymal cysts with an intrauterine neurotropic infection.[63] A subependymal cyst may occasionally be encountered on follow-up sonograms in conjunction with ventriculomegaly. The cyst may represent the residuum of a confined germinal matrix hematoma, the contralateral GMH having previously ruptured into the ventricular system, thereby providing a means for decompressing itself.

Because of the superficial location of the germinal matrix region, it is ideally evaluated using a high-resolution transducer. With routine 5.0-MHz scanning, it may occasionally be difficult to diagnose GMHs confidently. Follow-up of these hemorrhages has also improved with high resolution, and we have found that many of these hematomas develop multiple areas of internal cystic degeneration. This phase of maturation was not clearly visualized using lower frequency techniques; however, the internal septations seem to eventually degenerate, leading to the well-known unilocular subependymal cysts. All of the illustrations in this section were examples of 7.5-MHz scanning.

Grades II and III: Intraventricular Hemorrhage

Intraventricular hemorrhage (IVH) has received more attention than all other forms of neonatal intracranial pathology combined. There are many reasons for this, including its frequency, its association with PHH, and its often striking pathologic and radiographic appearance. The great attention given to IVH has, in fact, led many to ascribe this term inappropriately to almost any form of intracranial pathology that occurs in the premature neonate. The incorrect or imprecise use of such a specific pathologic or radiographic diagnosis should be strongly discouraged; an IVH implies bleeding into the ventricle and nothing more. Intraparenchymal or subependymal hemorrhage may be related, but these are really different entities and imply different immediate sequelae and prognoses. Needless to say, PVL is also different from IVH and is totally unrelated to the entire spectrum of GMRHs. The use of the term IVH should therefore be restricted to hemorrhage into the ventricular system. Furthermore, when referring to the generic types of intracranial hemorrhage, generic terms such as intracranial hemorrhage or CVH should be used, never the more specific diagnoses discussed above.

According to Pape and Wigglesworth, 95% of intraventricular hemorrhages in the premature are the result of transependymal rupture of a prior GMH.[8] Many authors support this contention,[10, 38, 64–66] but others report a high incidence of primary choroid plexus hemorrhage in prematures.[67–69] For example, Reeder[67] et al. described the choroid plexus as the origin of IVH in 59% of their patients. The true frequency of GMH versus choroid plexus hemorrhage is difficult to determine sonographically, because IVH of any kind often adheres to the choroid plexus.[64] We have, however, not infrequently found hemorrhage in the area of the choroid plexus in the presence of a normal germinal matrix. The actual site of origin of IVH is considerably more academic than practical. After Pape and Wigglesworth,[8] however, we shall assume that at least the majority of IVHs do originate in the germinal matrix.

Regardless of its origin, or where it is found

in the body, fresh hematoma is always brightly echogenic.[70-72] Blood seems rapidly transformed from its original anechoic, liquid state to a highly reflective clot. This transformation probably occurs as soon as blood coagulates and fibrin strands, red blood cells (RBCs), and other components form interfaces.

The actual physics of the change from anechoic to echogenic is relatively complicated. The reflectivity of any substance is directly related to its acoustic impedance, which in turn is dependent on only two variables, the speed of sound through a given medium and its density.[73] The former is the more important of the two, and various authors have demonstrated a considerable difference in the velocity of sound traveling through hematoma versus its velocity in either cerebrospinal fluid (CSF) or the neonatal brain.[74-76] Because the acoustic impedance of a hematoma is so much higher than that of the neonatal brain, the clot appears very echogenic. The hypoechoic brain and anechoic CSF provide excellent backgrounds with which to contrast the echogenicity of the hematoma. In vitro studies indicate that the velocity of sound through blood, and therefore its echogenicity, are dependent on hematocrit, the frequency of the transducer used, and the internal concentration of protein.[76-78]

We have termed the classic sonographic picture of a large IVH the "cast pattern".[24] The echogenic hematoma completely fills the ventricle and actually expands it. The hematoma seems to form a cast that conforms to the shape of the ventricle and solidifies. In some cases, the amount of intraventricular hematoma may be considerable; some neonates actually manifest a severe drop in their overall hematocrit from loss of blood in this manner. Most often the IVH is bilateral and fairly symmetric (Fig. 3-6, A and B). However, it may remain confined to one or the other ventricle. As illustrated in Fig. 3-6 A, the third ventricle may even be filled with blood. In this case, the ventricular cast may appear as a continuous echogenic Y-shaped structure on coronal sections, since hematoma in the foramina of Monro render them visible. Even if the hemorrhage originates from only one germinal matrix, it often accesses the entire ventricular system before organizing.[7] Leakage of blood beyond the ventricular system and into the subarachnoid space is also frequent,[8, 79] and probably contributes significantly to the development of PHH in many neonates (Fig. 3-6 C). Subarachnoid hemorrhage (SAH), although undoubtedly frequent in children with IVH, is poorly visualized by ultrasound, and to date no definite sonographic criteria for the adequate imaging of this entity have been laid down. SAH remains almost exclusively within the domain of the CT scanner.[4, 80]

Large echogenic blood casts are quite striking at sonography. On parasagittal sections, one can trace the entire distended ventricle including the frontal, occipital, and temporal horns. On the coronal sections alone, it may be difficult to confidently differentiate IVH from large subependymal hemorrhages, which produce a mass effect on the ventricles and obliterate them in the area of the frontal horn. However, if attention is directed posteriorly, the occipital horn will be visible and occupied by echogenic clot, confirming what is easily demonstrated in the parasagittal section. Blood is a fluid medium and fills an existing and expandable space; therefore, the borders of the hematoma should always be smooth. Because the hematoma is isoechoic to the choroid plexus, the two are usually inseparable sonographically. Recently, however, we seem to have increasing ability to separate hematoma from normal choroid. Whether this is dependent on timing or the use of higher resolution transducers is uncertain.

Large IVHs do not present diagnostic difficulties, but smaller hemorrhages can present considerable challenge. Fiske and co-workers[81] outlined a number of useful ways to help differentiate the normal choroid from small IVHs. The work of Bowie et al. describing the caudothalamic notch in detail is also useful in this regard,[59] and I will contribute a few ideas of my own on the subject. Practically speaking, there are cases where one is never sure whether the echogenicity is really caused by a large and sometimes irregular normal choroid plexus or by IVH. Luckily, the major concern in IVH is the development of significant PHH, and this is very rare following small hemorrhages. The follow-up scan in 1 week will show any ventriculomegaly that might have occurred. It will often actually show the hematoma to better advantage, for it may be suspended in anechoic CSF and not as closely adherent to the choroid plexus.

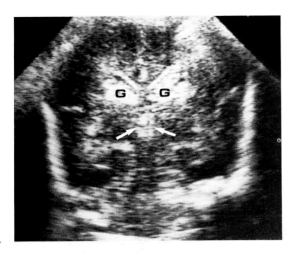

A

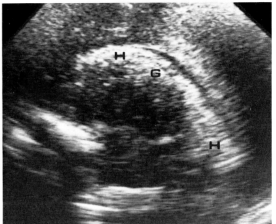

B

FIGURE 3-6. Large bilateral IVH, cast pattern. Homogeneously echogenic hematoma fills and expands both lateral ventricles. Cast is made up of both intraventricular (*H*) and germinal matrix (*G*) hematoma (**B**). Third ventricle (*arrows*) also contains hematoma, giving a Y-shaped appearance on coronal sections (**A**) Autopsy specimen (**C**) shows typical large, thick hematoma in basilar cisterns and around brain stem.

C

The surest method of confidently diagnosing IVH of any size is analysis of the anatomy of the normal choroid plexus (Fig. 3-7 A). The choroid plexus encircles the posterior thalamus and extends inferiorly into the temporal horn along with the fornix. It is largest in the area of the ventricular trigone (the glomus), and tapers as it rounds over the superoposterior thalamus. On the surface facing into the ventricle, the choroid should be relatively smooth. It should not extend into the occipital horn, although it is frequently bulbous in the area of the glomus. At the foramen of Monro, the choroid dives down into the third ventricle to lie in the midline. At this point, the choroid plexus forms the roof of the third ventricle and is known as the tela choroidea. If all neonates followed this pattern ex-

actly, differentiation between the normal and abnormal would be simple. Unfortunately, many neonates have a very large choroid plexus, often occupying almost the entire ventricle. In other normal neonates, it may extend into the occipital horn, and its surface may be rather irregular. Furthermore, it varies in size depending on gestational age. Knowledge of this normal anatomy will greatly aid the sonographer in the diagnosis of more subtle IVHs.

Drawing directly on the anatomy of the choroid, we find that any echogenic focus in the frontal horn surely represents hematoma, because the echogenic choroid plexus descends into the third ventricle through the foramen of Monro. The absence of choroidal tissue in the frontal horn is well known to neurosurgeons

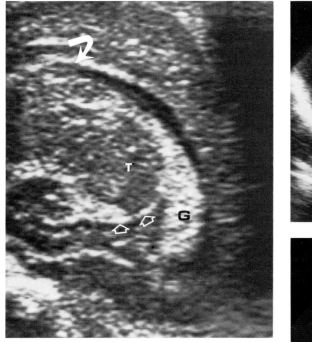

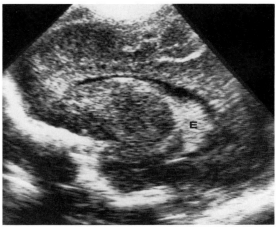

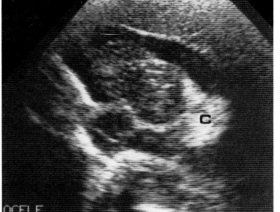

FIGURE 3-7. Normal choroid plexus versus small (Grade II) IVH. **A**, Normal choroid plexus surrounds the posterior thalamus (*T*) and has a smooth surface. Glomus (*G*) may appear as a separate structure from inferior fornix and extend for some distance into occipital horn (*open arrows*). Note absence of echogenicity in frontal horn (*curved arrow*).

B, Small IVH is manifested by "lumpiness" and mild enlargement of surface of choroid echo complex (*E*). **C**, Unusually prominent choroid plexus (*C*) in child with meningomyelocele. Although such bizarre configurations of the choroid plexus do not represent IVH in these children, they may be almost identical to it sonographically.

who optimally place the tips of shunt catheters there because it is devoid of choroid plexus.

Another useful method of differentiating between normal choroid plexus and adherent hematoma is through observing its contour in the region of the glomus (Fig. 3-7 B). An irregular or lumpy appearance is suggestive of hemorrhage. This lumpiness alone should be taken as a very soft finding in IVH; we have identified it in too many children who were normal. An example of the extreme variability of the choroid is found in children with congenital hydrocephalus associated with spinal dysraphism, where the normal choroidal glomus may be almost

masslike (Fig. 3-7 C). The reason for this is not certain, but it does not usually represent IVH in these children.[82]

A somewhat more definite diagnostic finding in smaller IVHs is the extension of the choroidal echo-complex into the occipital horn (Fig. 3-8 A). This probably represents IVH, and a repeat scan 1 week later will frequently show the hematoma to better advantage, because it is surrounded by CSF (Fig. 3-8 B). Again, we have seen normal choroid filling the occipital horn, and therefore this finding must also be considered rather soft.

A final method of diagnosing small IVHs that

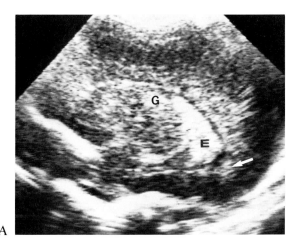
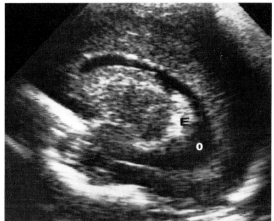

A

B

C

FIGURE 3-8. Abnormal choroid echo complex. **A,** choroid echo complex (*E*) extends too far into occipital horn; small focus of echogenicity (*arrow*) confirms diagnosis of IVH; it represents separate, dependent hematoma. Note GMH (*G*). Follow-up scan (**B**) in 2 weeks confirms original diagnosis of IVH. Note enlargement of occipital horn (*O*) and change in shape of choroid echo complex (*E*). **C,** Unusual section through posterior portion of skull shows fragment of hematoma (*H*) in the occipital horn (*arrows*) *C* = choroid plexus. Isolated chunks of hematoma are diagnostic of IVH.

are adherent to the choroid is found in the normal tapering of the choroid plexus as it rounds the superoposterior portion of the thalamus. As illustrated in Fig. 3-7 A, the choroid should gradually become thinner as it approaches the foramen of Monro. If it remains as thick as it was in the area of the glomus, a hemorrhage is probably present (Fig. 3-9 A). Again, this finding may require follow-up to prove or disprove the presence of hemorrhage. One pitfall should be mentioned in the diagnosis of smaller IVHs. When following the choroid plexus into the temporal horn it is normally accompanied by the inferior extension of the fornix. One may occasionally identify these as two separate structures in normal infants and be tempted to diagnose IVH; as illustrated in Fig. 3-7 A, however, the supposed clot is normal choroid plexus.

In diagnosing these small Grade II hemorrhages, one comforting fact can be kept in

mind. Small hemorrhages do not lead to significant PHH,[29, 36] and they have a very favorable outcome.[1, 20, 41, 42] In our own population, we found no significant difference in outcome when comparing children with normal cranial sonograms with those who had had GMHs or Grade II IVHs.[45] In this population, follow-up for PHH may be necessary for only a short time. Most importantly, clinicians and family can be assured that such small IVHs are of little if any clinical consequence. Such is not the case with large, Grade III IVHs; long periods of follow-up and frequent PHH should be anticipated. The paramount role of the sonographer in IVH, therefore, is in the diagnosis of large hematomas. Luckily, this is considerably simpler than diagnosing small ones.

The sequel specifically associated with IVH is PHH. Serial sonograms show that PHH can be identified as early as 1 or 2 days after the initial hemorrhagic event. Certainly within 2

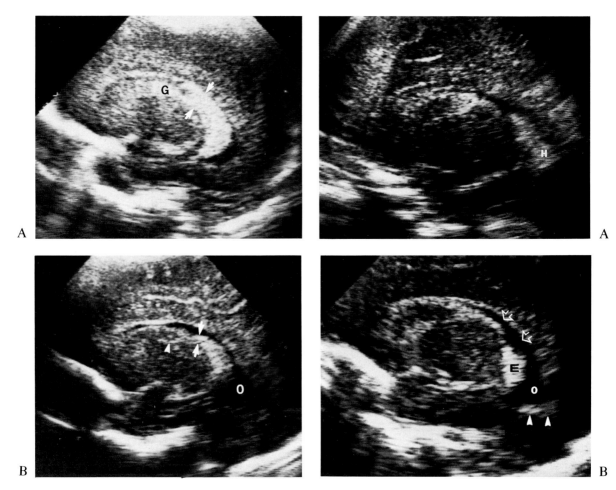

FIGURE 3-9. Nontapering of choroid echo complex representing IVH. **A**, Choroid echo complex remains wide (*arrows*) up to area of caudothalamic notch, suggesting IVH. Note GMH (*G*). Follow-up scan at 3 weeks (**B**) shows reversion of superior/ anterior portion of choroidal echo complex (*arrows*) to more normal tapered appearance and mild enlargement of occipital horn (*O*). GMH has also resolved, leaving only thin linear echogenicity (*arrowhead*).

FIGURE 3-10. Early PHH. (**A**), Small IVH (*H*) in posterior lateral ventricle. **B**, Follow-up scan at 1 week shows typical early PHH involving occipital horn (*O*) and superior portions of ventricular trigone (*open arrows*). Note that choroidal echo complex (*E*) has regained normal appearance. Small amount of dependent hematoma (*arrowheads*) persists.

weeks it should be evident if it is to ever be significant. In neonates with large IVHs, the hydrocephalus may worsen at an alarmingly rapid rate, and moderately severe ventriculomegaly may already be present within a few days. These children frequently develop intractable hydrocephalus and require protracted follow-up or even intervention.

The first parts of the ventricles to expand after hemorrhage are the superior trigones and the occipital horns[24, 83] (Fig. 3-10, A and B). In infants with small hemorrhages, these may be the only areas of the ventricles to ever enlarge. Following large hemorrhages, however, the entire lateral ventricle enlarges seemingly around the original castlike hematoma. Over time, the hematoma becomes smaller and disappears (Fig. 3-11, A–D). The time for this resorption is quite variable, but it is almost always completely accomplished by 5–6 weeks. While most hematomas fragment as they are being resorbed, some remain whole, and usually their centers become very hypoechoic or even anechoic. This picture may be confusing if the

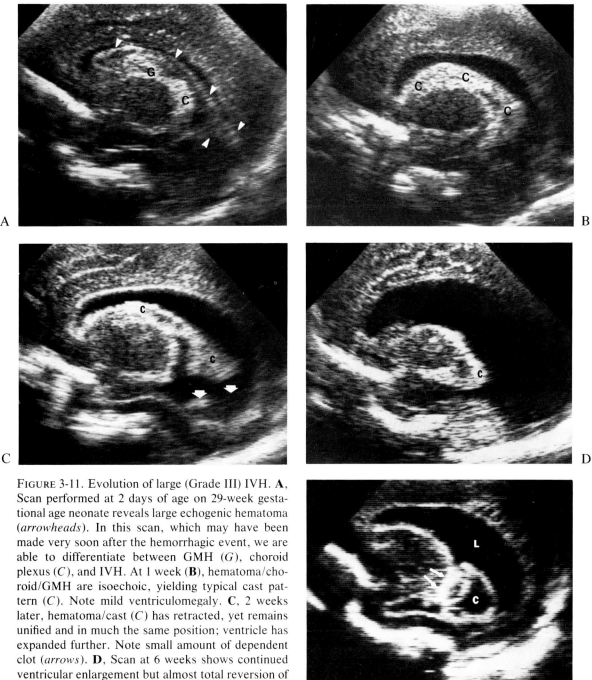

FIGURE 3-11. Evolution of large (Grade III) IVH. **A**, Scan performed at 2 days of age on 29-week gestational age neonate reveals large echogenic hematoma (*arrowheads*). In this scan, which may have been made very soon after the hemorrhagic event, we are able to differentiate between GMH (*G*), choroid plexus (*C*), and IVH. At 1 week (**B**), hematoma/choroid/GMH are isoechoic, yielding typical cast pattern (*C*). Note mild ventriculomegaly. **C**, 2 weeks later, hematoma/cast (*C*) has retracted, yet remains unified and in much the same position; ventricle has expanded further. Note small amount of dependent clot (*arrows*). **D**, Scan at 6 weeks shows continued ventricular enlargement but almost total reversion of choroidal echo complex to normal. Child had dramatic reversal of this worsening ventriculomegaly with institution of serial lumbar punctures. **E**, 6-week scan of different infant with large IVH. Single intraventricular hematoma has developed ventricular shape giving a "ventricle within a ventricle" appearance. *Arrows* point to choroid plexus. *L*, lateral ventricle. From Grant EG, Borts FT, Schellinger D, et al, 1981.[24]

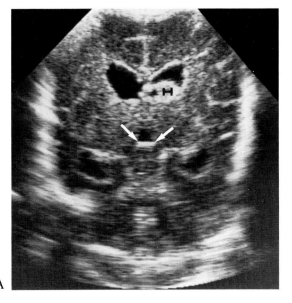

A

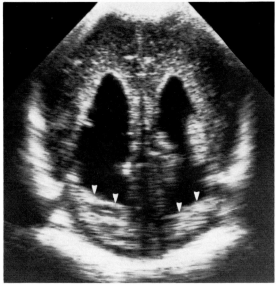

B

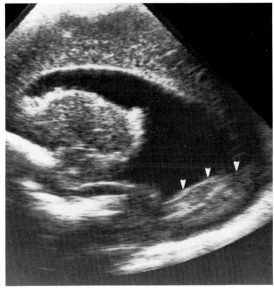

C

FIGURE 3-12. Cerebrospinal fluid/blood levels. Angled coronal (**A**), semiaxial (**B**), and parasagittal (**C**) sections reveal CSF/blood levels in occipital horns (*arrowheads*) and third ventricle (*arrows*). Hematoma at floor of frontal horn (*H*) in **A** probably represents posterior portion of germinal matrix hematoma or anterior part of intraventricular blood cast.

child was not scanned previously. It may actually appear that there is a "ventricle within a ventricle" (Fig. 3-11 D). This central anechoic area merely represents the normal maturation of the hematoma: The inner portions develop a gel-like consistency, while the outer portions form a sort of rind. This decreasing echogenicity within a hematoma is well known elsewhere in the body.[84] The unique feature of IVH is that it is surrounded by CSF, which sets up a particularly strong interface that causes the edge of the hematoma to appear especially bright and well defined.

Another feature of PHH is the formation of CSF/blood levels. Although some hematomas form casts and maintain a constant shape while being resorbed, others layer in the dependent portions of the ventricles. One may locate these levels in many places in the ventricles (Fig. 3-12, A and B), not necessarily the posterior portions. This probably occurs because, in contrast to a CT examination, we may move the baby from side to side, thus changing which part of the head is dependent. Although some authors have described movement of clot when observing with real-time scans, I cannot say I have ever convincingly observed this. Often when we follow a resolving hematoma, we find it in a consistent location within the ventricle on multiple examinations weeks apart. Hematoma can be detected sonographically in the ventricles for a relatively long while, frequently up to 6 weeks or more. This is a specific advantage of sonography over CT. CT requires increased density, and cannot consistently detect a hematoma that is more than 1–2 weeks old. For this reason, if PHH is suspected in a child in the absence of an early scan, sonography might confirm the presence of hematoma more accurately than CT.

Another common feature of PHH is ventricular asymmetry. One lateral ventricle is often larger than its counterpart. In some infants, one ventricle may be filled with hematoma while the opposite is markedly enlarged with CSF and contains no hematoma at all. In such cases it is often the ventricle without hematoma that enlarges most dramatically, while the ventricle filled with clot changes only minimally (Fig. 3-13, A and B).

To explain these unusual ventricular abnormalities, one must postulate the etiology of PHH to be multifactorial.[7, 20, 30, 79] Certainly, internal blockages caused by hematoma occluding narrow points in the ventricular system are a major factor. The occulusion of CSF flow at critical points such as the foramina of Monro, the aqueduct of Sylvius, or the points of egress of the CSF from the ventricles at the foramina of Luschka and Magendie could account for asymmetric ventricular expansion. Another factor in PHH is undoubtedly scarring of the arachnoid granulations. Such scarring results from an inflammatory arachnoiditis, which almost always accompanies significant SAH of any etiology,[86] and most neonates with large IVHs do extrude a sizeable amount of hematoma beyond the ventricles into the arachnoid space. Classically, as illustrated in Fig. 3-6 C, the blood that escapes from the ventricles forms a thick clot around the base of the brain. Blockage by hematoma alone may lead to focal ventriculomegaly, while scarring of the arachnoid granulations should result in panhydrocephalus. Any combination of these two major factors is possible and may lead to the varied ventricular abnormalities seen in PHH.

With PHH, the lateral ventricles are more

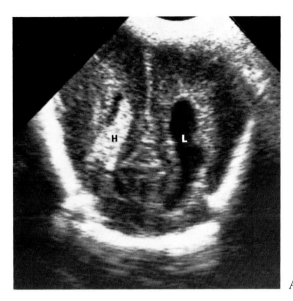

A

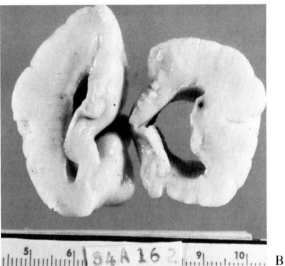

B

FIGURE 3-13. Semiaxial sonogram at 1 week of age (**A**) identifies large hematoma (*H*) filling right lateral ventricle. Left lateral ventricle (*L*) is enlarged by CSF. Child died 2 weeks later. Autopsy specimen (**B**) confirmed left ventricle is larger than right. Intervening sonograms revealed hematoma in right ventricle had almost completely resolved before death.

frequently and more severely affected than the third or fourth ventricles, respectively, and significant enlargement of the fourth ventricle is quite unusual.[87] This differential dilatation may be influenced by LaPlace's law in addition to blockage of the ventricles by hematoma. LaPlace's law states that as the radius of a cylinder (or any structure) increases, the forces of

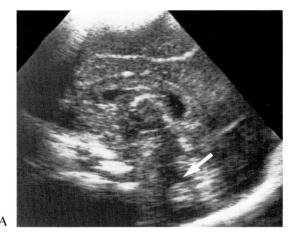

A

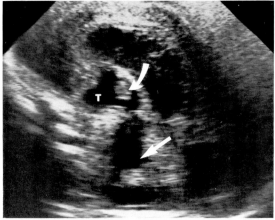

B

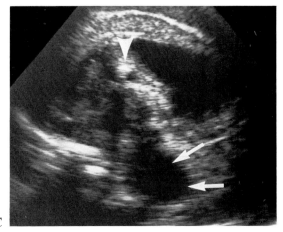

C

FIGURE 3-14. Posthemorrhagic enlargement of fourth ventricle. **A,** Normal fourth ventricle (*arrow*) at 2 days of age. Large IVH was discovered on scan at 7 days. **B,** Follow-up in 3 weeks shows mild enlargement of fourth ventricle (*arrow*), but massive dilatation of third (*T*) and lateral ventricles. Adherent clot causes massa intermedia to appear unusually large (*curved arrow*). Six-week scan (**C**) shows marked fourth ventricular enlargement after intervening bout of ventriculitis (*arrows*). Note shunt tip (*arrowhead*) in frontal horn.

pressure upon it increase as the square of the radius. Simply, the larger the structure, the more it will be affected by pressure and therefore the more it will tend to expand. The lateral ventricles are normally larger than the third ventricle, which is normally larger than the fourth. Similarly, the trigones and occipital horns of the lateral ventricles are normally the widest portions of these structures. The trigones and occipital horns are always the first portions of the ventricles to enlarge, and always the most severely affected by hydrocephalus. In even mild fourth ventricular enlargement, the lateral and third ventricles are always markedly dilated. Although massive posthemorrhagic enlargement of the fourth ventricle may occur, it has been quite unusual in our experience (Fig. 3–14, A and C). We did not see it at all in our early series of 172 neonates.[87] Overall, marked enlargement of the fourth ventricle occurred most frequently among our neonates who had IVH that was later complicated by ventriculitis. Although these infants did have significant PHH, it was not until the addition of ventriculitis that the hydrocephalus markedly affected the fourth ventricle.

An important point to be made concerning severe posthemorrhagic dilatation of the fourth ventricle is that on a single study it may appear similar to a Dandy–Walker malformation. PHH is not, however, congenital, unless one includes cases of intrauterine IVH. PHH usually follows hemorrhage and steadily worsening panventriculomegaly. In severe posthemorrhagic enlargement of the fourth ventricle, the lateral ventricles are huge. This is not typically the case in Dandy–Walker cyst, in which the lateral ventricles are usually proportionally smaller than the posterior fossa component. The vermis should also be absent in Dandy–Walker malformation, and classically one should identify a communication between a large fourth ventricle

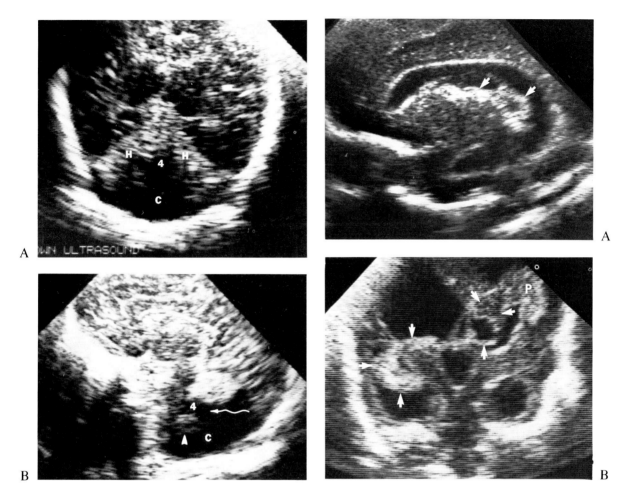

FIGURE 3-15. Dandy–Walker malformation. **A**, Fourth ventricle (*4*) is large. **B**, note communication (*curved arrow*) with extraaxial cyst (*C*) due to dysplastic inferior vermis (*arrowhead*). *H*, cerebellar hemisphere. (Reprinted with permission from Grant EG: Update on Neurosonography. In: Ultrasound Annual, 1984. Sanders RC, Hill M, eds. Raven Press, New York, 161–210, 1984.)

FIGURE 3-16. Intrauterine cerebroventricular hemorrhage: Both scans (**A** and **B**) were performed on first day of life. Large intraventricular hematomas (*arrows*) are present, but have a mature sonographic appearance and are accompanied by considerable PHH. Note intraparenchymal hemorrhage (*P*) in **B**.

and an extraaxial posterior fossa cyst (Fig. 3-15, A and B). In severe cases, however, only a single large cyst may be identified occupying almost the entire posterior fossa.[88, 89] The development of a severely dilated fourth ventricle in association with IVH and/or ventriculitis indicates that the situation is dire. Markedly increased intracranial pressure must be present, and, in spite of shunting, most of our neonates with marked enlargement of the fourth ventricle have died.

A brief discussion of intrauterine IVH is ger-

mane at this point. Until very recently, intrauterine IVH was unknown. With increasing use of prenatal sonography and increased awareness of CVH, however, reports of this condition have begun to appear in the literature.[90–93] Most of the neonates reported were born alive.[91–93] We have occasionally encountered neonates who appeared to have had intrauterine IVH. These infants have mature intraventricular hematoma and mild to severe hydrocephalus at birth (Fig. 3-16, A and B). Intrauterine CVH seems logical, since the fetus does have a germinal matrix before 32 weeks gestational age. Children examined during the first days of life who are found to have hydrocephalus and obviously mature clots in the ventricles should be diagnosed as having had intrauterine IVH. They should then be followed to assess the course of PHH in the same manner as any other neonate.

In addition to knowledge of the basic appearance of IVH and PHH, the sonographer must have knowledge of their treatment in order to be an adequate consultant. Again, a familiarity with the normal situation must precede the ability to diagnose the abnormal. The "normal" situation in this case is the child with IVH who develops PHH and has no intervention. PHH, whether mild or severe, follows a typical course consisting of ventricular expansion, stabilization, and, most frequently, a return to normal. In some cases, the hydrocephalus may be massive and rapid in onset. In others, ventriculomegaly may only be fleeting and mild.[94-96] As we have already discussed, PHH is very dependent on the size of the original hemorrhage.

Serial studies show that almost all neonates have at least some degree of ventricular enlargement following a hemorrhage. In small IVHs, ventriculomegaly may actually be totally resolved by the time of a routine scan in 7 days. Even following a relatively large IVH, many neonates eventually return to normal or near normal (Fig. 3-17, A–D); less than 5% of our own neonates have required shunts. Although some institutions advocate a much more aggressive approach,[97, 98] most seem convinced at present that PHH is usually self-limited, reserving shunting for only the most extreme cases.[95] Why the ventricles expand and eventually stabilize is only speculation. The choroid plexus produces a constant amount of CSF daily, and if it has no method of egress of resorption, the ventricles must enlarge. Perhaps the scarring, synechia, or hematoma that are responsible for the CSF accumulation eventually break down, restoring more normal CSF dynamics.

It is not unusual to find persistent, mild ventriculomegaly after large IVHs if these children are followed. The significance of this mild ventriculomegaly, if any, may take years to assess adequately. Many infants will also exhibit considerable asymmetry when the left and right lateral ventricles are compared after IVH (Fig. 3-17 E). To date, however, no one has attached much significance to these minimal abnormali-

ties. The major concern with minimal PHH is, of course, that it could represent ex vacuuo hydrocephalus, implying cerebral atrophy. Using animal models, some authors have shown that hydrocephalus alone can cause cerebral damage.[99,100] Other researchers have not corroborated this in humans.[101]

Extensive follow-up studies on children are imperative if the eventual meaning of small degrees of PHH is ever to be known. Much research will undoubtedly be directed toward the interactions of brain, hemorrhage, and hydrocephalus in the future. Newer imaging modalities such as magnetic resonance imaging (MRI) promise to be particularly exciting in this regard, and may offer further insight into the complex pathology of the neonatal brain. MRI has recently shown abnormal areas about the hydrocephalic ventricles in children,[102] but only limited work has been directed toward this problem in neonates. Our own follow-up of neonates with sometimes severe PHH is optimistic, and the majority of our children with even large IVHs have done quite well.

While most children with IVH experience the routine course of hemorrhage, ventriculomegaly, and the return to normal, some undergo progressive ventricular enlargement. The ventricles never stabilize, and eventually the neonate reaches a situation we have come to call "intractable hydrocephalus." The decision to institute therapy for this progressive ventricular expansion is a difficult one, and requires close contact between the radiologist and the clinician.

At our institution, serial lumbar punctures are generally the first form of treatment attempted; Drug therapy has never been popular among our neonatologists. The actual effectiveness of serial lumbar punctures in treating PHH remains quite controversial. If blockage of CSF egress from the ventricles plays any etiologic role in PHH, one must seriously question why they should have any effect at all. Papile et al. have reported success,[103] and Mantovani et al. failure,[104] of serial lumbar punctures to control hydrocephalus. The obvious difficulty with any study assessing the success of serial lumbar punctures in treating PHH lies again in its natural history. Are we temporizing and are these children getting better on their own, or does this

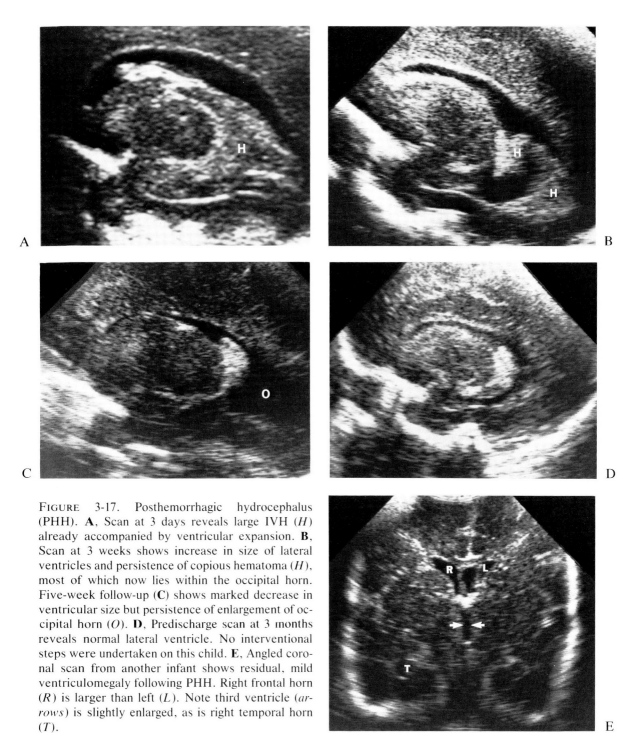

FIGURE 3-17. Posthemorrhagic hydrocephalus (PHH). **A**, Scan at 3 days reveals large IVH (*H*) already accompanied by ventricular expansion. **B**, Scan at 3 weeks shows increase in size of lateral ventricles and persistence of copious hematoma (*H*), most of which now lies within the occipital horn. Five-week follow-up (**C**) shows marked decrease in ventricular size but persistence of enlargement of occipital horn (*O*). **D**, Predischarge scan at 3 months reveals normal lateral ventricle. No interventional steps were undertaken on this child. **E**, Angled coronal scan from another infant shows residual, mild ventriculomegaly following PHH. Right frontal horn (*R*) is larger than left (*L*). Note third ventricle (*arrows*) is slightly enlarged, as is right temporal horn (*T*).

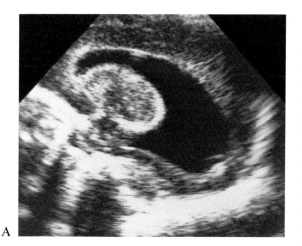

A

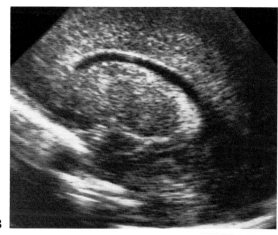

B

FIGURE 3-18. Success of serial lumbar punctures. Steadily worsening PHH (**A**) at 5 weeks decreases dramatically (**B**) after 1 week of serial lumbar punctures.

treatment actually work? Levene and Starte[95] point out that their "success" without treatment was very similar to that reported by Papile[103] using serial lumbar puncture. At present we do institute such therapy, and it has occasionally produced seemingly dramatic results (Fig. 3-18, A and B).

In those unusual cases where both nature and serial lumbar punctures have failed to reverse steadily worsening PHH, the final option is a shunt. Before resorting to an internalized ventriculoperitoneal or ventriculoatrial shunt, many would utilize a simple "reservoir." A reservoir is a tube placed into the ventricle that extends to a pouch beneath the scalp. A needle

is inserted to draw off excess CSF. This process is repeated until the amount of CSF withdrawn decreases. When continued taps fail to produce fluid, a sonogram should be performed to assure that the ventricles are of normal size. This decrease in ventricular size may be quite dramatic, and the ventricles sometimes return to normal size in as little as a week (Fig. 3-19, A and B). In other infants, considerable quantities of CSF may be withdrawn for up to several months. This latter, protracted course is fortunately very unusual. With continued minimal return from the reservoir and a sonogram confirming that the entire ventricular system has decompressed, withdrawal of CSF may be discontinued. At this juncture, follow-up sonography in perhaps 2 or 3 weeks is essential to ensure that PHH has not recurred.

The sonographer obviously plays a major role both in the decision to institute therapy and in following its effectiveness. Almost all decisions based on the sonographic assessment of hydrocephalus depend on the comparison of serial sonograms. Therefore, one must scan with attention to reproducible results. Frequently, measurements at the midportions of the bodies of the lateral ventricles have been used for this purpose.[30, 95, 105, 106] Although this method has a few shortcomings, it is probably the most easily reproduced dimension of the lateral ventricles and a practical area of measure. One must keep in mind that the entire ventricular system is involved in PHH, and a measurement or at least a visual assessment of the trigone/occipital horn can sometimes add another helpful parameter.

We depend less and less on absolute measurements, preferring rather to observe changes in ventricular contour, with particular attention to the frontal horns. Because the frontal horns are always the least affected portions of the lateral ventricles in hydrocephalus, they are most easily evaluated. The frontal horns are always surrounded by some cortical mantle in PHH. They are usually easily defined on a single section, both in the coronal and parasagittal orientations. On parasagittal sections, pointing of the anterior tip of the frontal horn that has given way to rounding provides an easy monitor of ventricular enlargement (Fig. 3-20, A and B). Similarly, outward bulging of the inferolateral

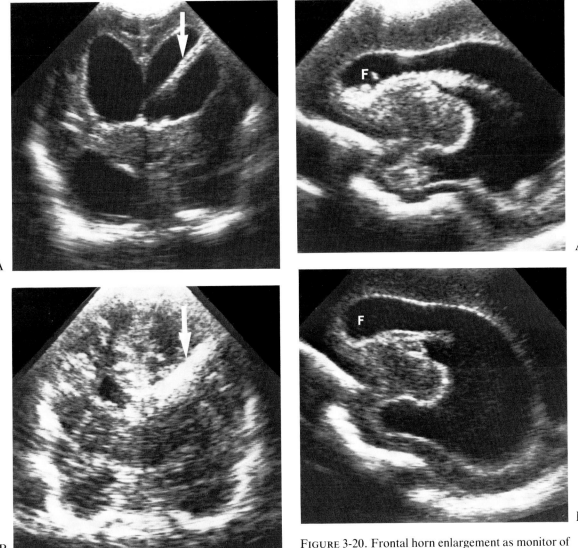

A

B

FIGURE 3-19. Insertion of reservoir: Shunt tip (*arrow*) (**A** and **B**) in left lateral ventricle of child with intractable hydrocephalus. **B**, 1 week later, ventricles are almost normal size.

FIGURE 3-20. Frontal horn enlargement as monitor of ventricular distension: Both scans reveal marked enlargement of right lateral ventricle after large IVH. **A** was performed 1 week before **B**. Posterior portions of lateral ventricle are difficult to assess for change in size. Frontal horn (*F*) appears more tense and has developed a bulbous, rounded contour indicating ventricle has enlarged.

border of the frontal horn on coronal sections indicates increasing ventricular size.

This extensive discussion of PHH is included because it is the typical sequel to IVH. Although many studies equate the outcome of the child to the original hemorrhagic event, it is the evaluation of ventricular enlargement that consumes so much of the neurosonographer's time. A complete discussion of IVH therefore de-

mands a detailed description of the many aspects of PHH.

Grade IV: Intraparenchymal Hemorrhage

Cerebral intraparenchymal hemorrhage (IPH) may refer to any form of bleeding into the substance of the brain. In the context of the preterm infant, however, our definition of IPH must be very specific, for its sequelae are also specific, both sonographically and with regard to clinical outcome. At sonography, a unilocular, focal, porencephalic cyst will eventually replace the area of the original cerebral hematoma in all cases of IPH.[37-40] Clinically, among all the forms of hemorrhage originating in the germinal matrix, IPH has the poorest prognosis and is associated with the most severe neurologic deficits.[41, 42] For our purposes, IPH may be defined as hemorrhage into the substance of the brain that has originated in the germinal matrix and extended into the cerebral parenchyma beyond the confines of that structure.

Many other forms of cerebral IPH may occur in preterm infants: hemorrhage secondary to birth trauma, ruptured arteriovenous malformation, or Rh isoimmunization, to name a few. Although these hemorrhages are also into the parenchyma of the brain, by our definition they belong in a separate category; they do not originate in the germinal matrix. They result from a variety of different processes that are not at all associated with gestational immaturity. The differentiation of germinal matrix-related IPH from other forms of cerebral IPH is, however, quite important. More invasive procedures may be warranted; for example, if arteriovenous malformation is suspected. In other forms of IPH, surgical evacuation of the hematoma may be necessary. Germinal matrix-related IPH, on the other hand, is treated conservatively; no one has yet attempted surgical intervention in this lesion.

A brief note should also be added about the differences between IPH and PVL. Both affect the area of the brain directly adjacent to the lateral ventricles. PVL also may have a component of IPH, but it does not originate in the germinal matrix. Hemorrhage into PVL is actually secondary to an earlier infarction. PVL has a different etiology, a different sonographic appearance, both acutely and in follow-up, and even different prognostic implications from the intraparenchymal or Grade IV hemorrhage discussed in this section.

Earlier in this chapter we described the sonographic features of isolated GMH and its most common form of extension, IVH. Spread of GMH may also proceed along other lines, and it

may dissect into the cerebral parenchyma. Because IVH is much more frequent than IPH, one must postulate that the ependyma is more easily violated than the substance of the brain. Factors other than mere size or pressure of a GMH may actually be responsible for IPH. Increased permeability of the brain due to an earlier injury (ischemia, perhaps) might facilitate the spread of a GMH into the parenchyma. If ischemia were actually involved, IPH would be etiologically much closer in its origin to the hemorrhage that often accompanies PVL.

The sonographic features of IPH are all closely related to its germinal matrix origin. The hallmark of IPH is the identification of a brightly echogenic masslike area adjacent to the lateral ventricle. Recent hematoma is usually ragged but well defined at its borders, with a homogeneous internal echo pattern. Because IPH originates in the germinal matrix, it is most frequently found in the frontoparietal regions (Fig. 3-21 A). This feature is most apparent in small-to-moderate-sized IPHs. At times, IPHs may be so extensive that they involve much of one or the other cerebral hemisphere, extending in some cases almost to the surface of the brain (Fig. 3-21 B). The focal origins of these large hemorrhages will, therefore, often be obscured.

IPH is always accompanied by IVH, again harkening back to the premise that the ependyma is more easily penetrated than is healthy parenchyma. Another explanation for the constant association of IVH and IPH, however, is offered by Larroche.[79] She ascribes IPH to a disruption of the ependyma of the corner of the lateral ventricle, which leads to a necrotic-hemorrhagic lesion of the underlying white matter. Regardless of the reason, because IPH and IVH always occur together and are isoechoic, the typical picture of IPH is one of a large, continuous, ventricular blood cast that extends beyond the anticipated location of the ependyma and out into the parenchyma. The choroid plexus, it will be remembered, is also isoechoic when compared to intraventricular hematoma, and these three components combine to form an extensive, homogeneous echo complex.[107] This echo complex results in the striking sonographic picture so frequently associated with IPH (Fig. 3-22, A and B).

Another sonographic feature of IPH is "mass effect"; one often finds contralateral deviation

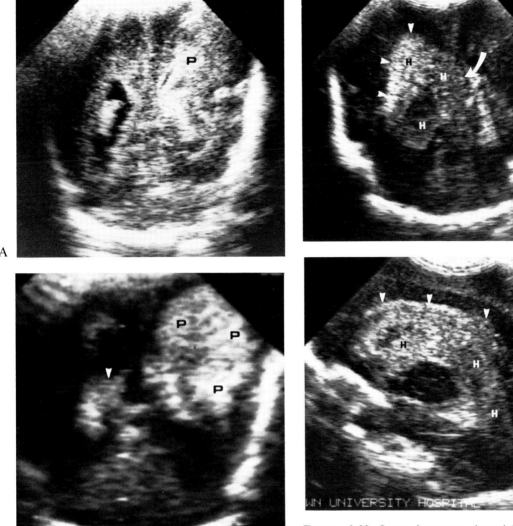

A

B

A

B

FIGURE 3-21. Intraparenchymal hemorrhage (IPH). **A**, Small parenchymal hematoma (*P*) is focal and in proximity of germinal matrix, therefore frontoparietal location is essential. **B**, Focal nature may be obscured in large parenchymal hemorrhage (*P*). Much of left frontoparietal lobes are involved, and hematoma extends to almost to surface of the brain. Note CSF/blood level in right lateral ventricle (*arrowhead*).

FIGURE 3-22. Large intraparenchymal hemorrhage (IPH). Axial (**A**) and right parasagittal (**B**) sections reveal large right IPH (*arrowheads*), which forms a continuous echo complex (*H*) with IVH and choroid plexus. Note masslike extension of hematoma across midline (*curved arrow*).

of the midline structures in the area of the hemorrhage (Fig. 3-23 A). Depending on the extent and location of the hematoma, the ipsilateral Sylvian fissure may be depressed as well (Fig. 3-23 B). This mass effect forms part of the sonographic constellation of findings in IPH; it is not

present in PVL. This difference in these two forms of intracranial pathology lends credence to the premise that GMRH is caused by bleeding under pressure, while PVL is the result of infarction.

The sonographic diagnosis of IPH is usually straightforward. In some cases, however, the differentiation between hematoma confined to the ventricle and hematoma adjacent to it may present considerable challenge. This is especially so in smaller IPHs and in cases where the

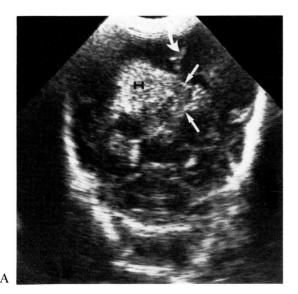

A

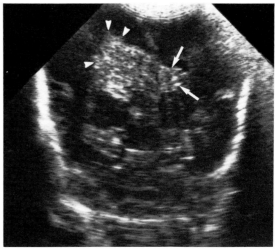

FIGURE 3-24. Comparison of IPH (*arrowheads*) with IVH (*arrows*). The former has very ragged edges, while the latter is quite smooth in contour.

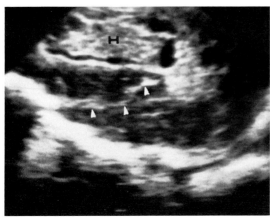

B

FIGURE 3-23. Mass effect and IPH. **A**, Large right intraparenchymal hematoma (*H*) extends across midline (*arrows*) and causes marked contralateral deviation of the falx/interhemispheric fissure (*curved arrow*). **B** shows inferior displacement of Sylvian fissure (*arrowheads*) by maturing intraparenchymal hematoma (*H*), which is surrounded by CSF as porencephalic cyst forms.

ventricles are greatly distended by blood. Comparison of the right and left frontal horns on a coronal section may occasionally be of assistance in equivocal cases (Fig. 3-24 A). With IPH, one finds a focal, asymmetric outpouching of echogenicity that is not present on the opposite side. The echogenicity of IVH is also sharply and smoothly defined, whereas IPH may have a more ragged border; IPH is not con-

fined by the ependyma. At times, scanning from various angles may show IPH to better advantage. One properly angled section may demonstrate a distinct outpouching of increased echogenicity that definitely extends beyond the ventricle. IPH may also appear more obvious after the onset of PHH and maturation of the original hematoma. In these cases, follow-up scans may show the extraventricular nature of an IPH to best advantage. Finally, one may have to use the eventual development of a porencephalic cyst as confirmation of the original IPH.

Like other forms of GMH, IPH has a typical sequel, porencephaly. Earlier authors have attributed porencephaly to a host of insults ranging from intrauterine anoxia or infection to needle puncture for ventriculography.[109-111] Although various factors may be involved when considering etiology of all porencephaly, many of the cases of "congenital porencephaly" found later in life are undoubtedly the result of neonatal IPH. Intrauterine IPH has also recently been described. Chinn and Filly[91] reported a neonate born with hydrocephalus and a partially mature IPH/porencephalic cyst; the appearance of the hematoma indicated that the original hemorrhage occurred in utero. The recently discovered connection between perinatal

IPH and porencephaly implies that, indeed, many cases of porencephaly discovered later in life may have had their origin in an early IPH.

Porencephaly follows IPH in every instance,[37-40] and we have found a direct correlation between the size of the original hemorrhage and the eventual size of the porencephalic cyst.[37] Small IPHs lead to small areas of porencephaly, and large parenchymal hemorrhages lead to large cerebral defects (Fig. 3-25, A and B). The progression from IPH to porencephaly is somewhat akin to the findings of IVH as it matures. The original IPH is intensely and homogeneously echogenic. Over a relatively short period of time (a few days to 2 weeks), the inner portions of the hematoma become hypoechoic. The outer borders remain highly echogenic and become sharply demarcated from the surrounding cerebral parenchyma. We have termed this the "rind phase." Pathologically, the inner portions of the hematoma undergo liquefaction and become progressively more anechoic. The outer borders, meanwhile, form a more solid, echogenic "rind" at the interface with the cerebral tissue. A similar picture of a maturing hematoma with echogenic borders and an anechoic or hypoechoic center has already been described in the ventricle. Following the "rind phase," the hematoma becomes progressively smaller and undergoes "clot retraction."

It is during this retraction period that the developing cyst can first be identified. As the clot retracts, it leaves behind a cerebral defect that is a perfect cast of the original hematoma and occupied by anechoic CSF. In many instances a large intraparenchymal/intraventricular hematoma complex will remain. The two may stay attached and be resorbed together, or may fragment and undergo retraction/resorption separately. Eventually, the parenchymal clot resolves entirely, leaving behind a porencephalic cyst in direct communication with the lateral ventricle (Figs. 26 A–D). Although the progression from IPH to porencephaly is fairly orderly, the time sequence is not. Among our patients, complete formation of the porencephalic cyst varied from 2 weeks to 60 days after the initial event.

The size of the porencephalic cyst may be directly dependent on the size of the original IPH; however, the effect of coexistent hydro-

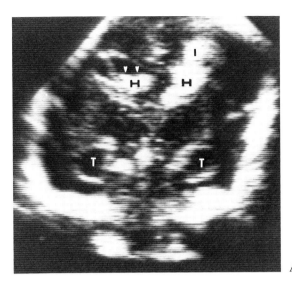

A

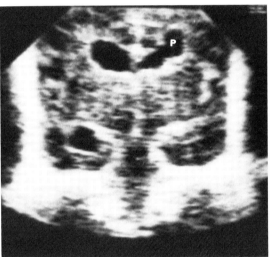

B

FIGURE 3-25. Small, focal IPH. **A**, Coronal section at 3 days of age reveals small left IPH (*I*) accompanied by bilateral IVH (*H*) and early enlargement of right frontal horn and temporal horns (*T*). Note CSF/blood level on right (*arrowheads*). **B**, Follow-up at 8 weeks reveals left porencephalic cyst (*P*) of approximately same size as original hematoma.

cephalus and CSF pressure on a porencephalic cyst may be considerable. A few specific cases illustrate this point nicely. One neonate suffered a small IPH and developed a correspondingly small area of porencephaly. Because of intractable hydrocephalus, a shunt was eventually required. The ventricles rapidly returned to normal size, and the small porencephalic cyst was no longer identified at sonography. This

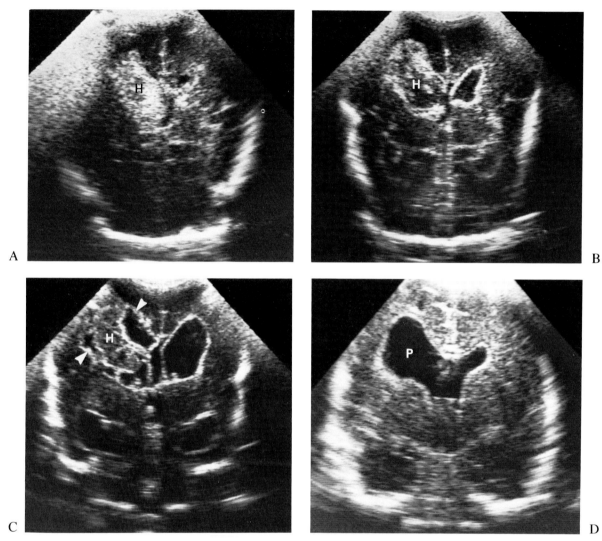

FIGURE 3-26. Evolution from IPH to porencephalic cyst. Angled coronal section at 3 days (**A**) reveals large right IPH/IVH (*H*). Note homogeneously echogenic appearance. At 2 weeks (**B**), maturing hematoma (*H*) has developed echogenic borders and hypoechoic center—"rind phase." **C**, 4-week scan shows "clot retraction"; hematoma (*H*) decreases in size, leaving behind a large CSF-filled cerebral defect (*arrowheads*). **D**, 8-week scan reveals mature porencephalic cyst (*P*). Both cyst and ventricles have decreased in size; ventricular reservoir was inserted at 6 weeks.

same infant later developed shunt failure and reexpansion of the ventricles; a sonogram revealed a reappearance of the porencephalic cyst at that time (Fig. 3-27, A–C).

Another child with a large right IPH developed a large right frontoparietal porencephalic cyst. Marked PHH accompanied the porencephaly and shunting was undertaken. Similar to the first child, the ventricles decompressed. The large right frontoparietal defect, however, remained although somewhat decreased in size (Fig. 3-28). The changes in the size of the porencephalic cysts imply direct communication between the cysts and the ventricles. Other interesting points about IPH/porencephaly may also be taken from these two cases. In the first case, the cyst disappeared with ventricular decompression. Reappearance of the cyst with shunt failure, however, implied that although we may no longer identify the cyst, a cerebral defect

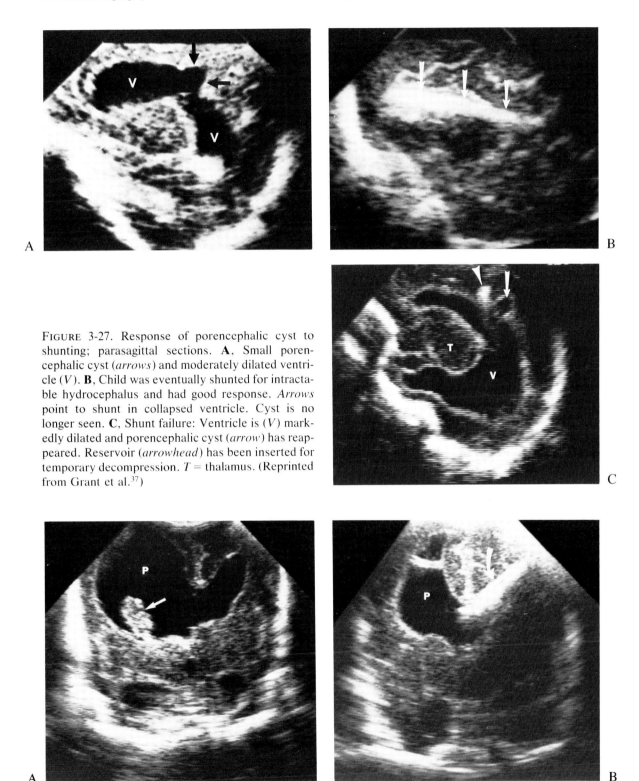

FIGURE 3-27. Response of porencephalic cyst to shunting; parasagittal sections. **A**, Small porencephalic cyst (*arrows*) and moderately dilated ventricle (*V*). **B**, Child was eventually shunted for intractable hydrocephalus and had good response. *Arrows* point to shunt in collapsed ventricle. Cyst is no longer seen. **C**, Shunt failure: Ventricle is (*V*) markedly dilated and porencephalic cyst (*arrow*) has reappeared. Reservoir (*arrowhead*) has been inserted for temporary decompression. *T* = thalamus. (Reprinted from Grant et al.[37])

FIGURE 3-28. Response of porencephalic cyst to shunting. **A**, Huge right porencephalic cyst (*P*) causes midline deviation and is accompanied by severe ventricular enlargement. Note residual hematoma (*arrow*). **B**, Following insertion of reservoir (*curved arrow*), ventricles are decompressed; although it is somewhat decreased in size, the cyst remains quite large.

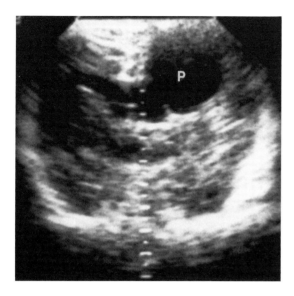

FIGURE 3-29. Coronal section in an 18-month-old child with a history of IPH/porencephaly at 3 days of age shows persistence of porencephalic cyst (*P*) although ventricles are only moderately enlarged. Child had no interventional procedures. At 3 years of age, she is paraplegic.

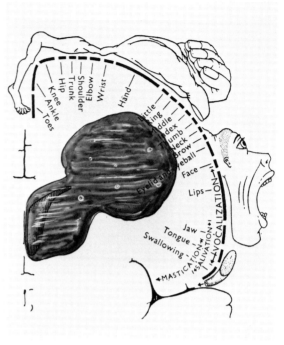

FIGURE 3-30. Homunculus with superimposition of porencephalic cyst shows possible relationship of cerebral defect to essential motor areas of brain.

remains that may not be sonographically visible. The second case illustrates a more distressing situation; the ventricles decreased in size following the shunt, yet the cyst remained. In this case, although the increased CSF pressure was relieved, there was simply not enough cerebral tissue remaining to fill the void.

Similarly, in another child who never required intervention, a follow-up sonogram performed 18 months after the diagnosis of IPH/porencephaly showed relatively normal-sized ventricles but persistence of the cerebral defect (Fig. 3-29). We have also identified a number of neonates who developed cerebral atrophy after IVH/IPH. Although IPH appears to be a focal lesion, one must question if these children actually suffered a severe and generalized cerebral insult that allowed the development of IPH.

The clinical results in children with IPH have been varied, but overall, they are the worst among neonates with GMRH. Children with small lesions may do well in our experience. Children with large IPHs and resultant large areas of porencephaly generally do poorly. A review of the homunculus may partially explain this (Fig. 3-30). Many important functional areas of cerebral tissue may be destroyed in a large IPH, and the possibility of other areas of the developing brain assuming their function seems doubtful.

Before leaving the subject of intracranial hemorrhage for periventricular leukomalacia (PVL), a brief discussion of cerebellar hemorrhage will be included. The pathology literature indicates that 15–25% of preterm neonates have cerebellar hemorrhage.[112-115] Pape and Wigglesworth also described cerebellar hemorrhage as common[8], yet we have identified only one in our entire population. This, of course, may say more about our scanning than the frequency of cerebellar hemorrhage in the preterm neonate. A review of the sonographic and CT literature, however, vindicates our scanning technique and would support the contention that in life, cerebellar hemorrhage is quite rare.[116-120]

A plausible explanation for the discrepancy between the radiographic and autopsy frequency of the lesion may be that many autopsy lesions were microscopic, while the cerebellar hemorrhages described thus far in the literature

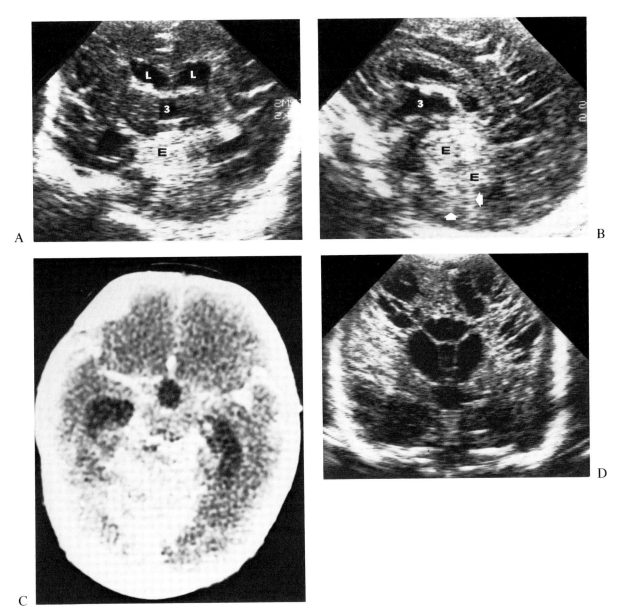

FIGURE 3-31. Cerebellar hemorrhage. Angled coronal (**A**) and midline sagittal (**B**) sections reveal large echogenic focus (*E*) in posterior fossa that extends into area of quadrigeminal plate. Normal cerebellar tissue can be identified inferiorly (*arrows*). Third (*3*) and lateral (*L*) ventricles are enlarged. **C**, CT scan confirms hemorrhagic nature of lesion and defines large subarachnoid component. **D**, Follow-up scan at 1 month with conservative treatment shows the development of diffuse cystic encephalomalacia. The latter abnormality may have been secondary to diffuse vascular spasm associated with subarachnoid hemorrhage.

have been quite large. Another possibility is that most of the children with cerebellar hemorrhage do not survive; therefore, in many cases it could represent a preterminal event that is not frequently imaged in the living neonate. Foy et al.[116] raise the possibility that some cerebellar hemorrhages may be masked; however, Foy described the cerebellar hemispheres as having relatively high echogenicity. In our experience, the cerebellar hemispheres are of low-level echogenicity[87] and therefore should not mask hemorrhage. Although the cerebellar vermis is brightly echogenic, I must presume that a hemorrhage small enough to hide in that structure would probably be very difficult to see even if it was contrasted by surrounding hypoechoic tissues.

Cerebellar hemorrhage does occur in the preterm infant and can be successfully identified by ultrasound (Fig. 3-31, A–D). In the few reported cases, it was as echogenic as IPH in other areas of the brain.[116–119] Although these hemorrhages can apparently be devastating, I must continue to question their actual frequency in the living patient because so little has been written about them. Cerebellar hemorrhage deserves more attention in the future, and even the treatment remains controversial; like its supratentorial counterpart, conservative management seems the usual method of treatment in the premature.[120, 121]

References

1. Burstein J, Papile L, Burstein R. Intraventricular hemorrhage and hydrocephalus in premature newborns: A prospective study with CT. AJR 132:631–635, 1979.
2. Cartwright GW, Culbertson K, Schreiner RL, Garg BP. Changes in clinical presentation of term infants with intracranial hemorrhage. Dev Med Child Neurol 21:730–737, 1979.
3. Scher MS, Wright FS, Lockman LA, Thompson TR. Intraventricular hemorrhage in the full-term neonate. Arch Neurol 39:769–772, 1982.
4. Siegel MJ, Patel J, Gado MH, Shackelford GD. Cranial computed tomography and real-time sonography in full-term neonates and infants. Radiology 149:111–116, 1983.
5. Volpe J. Neonatal intracranial hemorrhage: pathophysiology, neuropathology and clinical features. Clin Perinatol 4:77–102, 1977.
6. Grant EG, Schellinger D, Grosso MA, Jacobs NM, Richardson JD. Intracranial hemorrhage in neonates with erythroblastosis fetalis: Sonographic and CT findings. AJNR 5:259–262, 1984.
7. Wigglesworth JS, Pape KE. Pathophysiology of intracranial haemorrhage in the newborn. J Perinat Med 8:119–133, 1980.
8. Pape KE, Wigglesworth JE. Haemorrhage, Ischemia and the Perinatal Brain. Lippincott, Philadelphia, 1979.
9. Fedrick J, Butler NR. Certain causes of neonatal death. II. Intraventricular hemorrhage. Biol Neonate 15:257–290, 1970.
10. Leech RW, Kohmen P. Subependymal and intraventricular hemorrhage in the newborn. Am J Pathol 77:465–476, 1974.
11. Farwell JR, Scott DT. Fatal intracranial hemorrhage in prematures: Findings at autopsy in 80 consecutive cases. Pediatr Res 13:524, 1979.
12. Levene MI, Wigglesworth JS, Dubowitz V. Cerebral structure and intraventricular haemorrhage in the neonate: A real-time ultrasound study. Arch Dis Child 56:416–424, 1981.
13. Cooke RWI. Factors associated with periventricular haemorrhage in very low birthweight infants. Arch Dis Child 56:425–431, 1981.
14. Smith WL, McGuinness G, Cavanaugh D, Courtney S. Ultrasound screening of premature infants: Longitudinal follow-up of intracranial hemorrhage. Radiology 147:445–448, 1983.
15. Callen PW. Ultrasonography in Obstetrics and Gynecology. Saunders, Philadelphia, 1983.
16. Sanders RC, James AE. The Principles and Practice of Ultrasonography in Obstetrics and Gynecology. Appleton-Century-Crofts, New York, 1980.
17. Dubowitz LMS, Dubowitz V, Goldberg C. Clinical assessment of gestational age in the newborn infant. J Pediatr 77:1–10, 1970.
18. Tsiantos A, Victorin L, Relier JP, Dyer N, Sundell H, Brill AB, Stahlman M. Intracranial hemorrhage in the prematurely born infant. J Pediatr 85:854–859, 1974.
19. Cole VA, Durbin GM, Olaffson A, Reynolds EOR, Rivers RPA, Smith JF. Pathogenesis of intraventricular hemorrhage in newborn infants. Arch Dis Child 49:722–728, 1974.
20. Pape KE. Intraventricular hemorrhage: Diagnosis and outcome. Birth Defects 13:143–151, 1981.
21. Lazzara A, Shumann PA, Dykes F, Bramm AW, Schwartz J. Clinical predictability of intraventricular hemorrhage in pre-term infants. Pediatrics 65:30–34, 1980.
22. Bejar R, Curbelo V, Coen RW, Leopold G, James H, Gluck L. Diagnosis and follow-up of intraventricular and intracerebral hemorrhages by ultrasound studies of infant's brain through the fontanelles and sutures. Pediatrics 66:661–673, 1980.
23. Lee BP, Grassi AE, Schechner S, Auld PAM. Neonatal intraventricular hemorrhage: A serial computed tomography study. J Comput Assist Tomogr 3:483–490, 1979.
24. Grant EG, Borts FT, Schellinger D, McCullough D, Sirasulramanian KN, Smith Y. Real-time ultrasonography of neonatal intraventricular hemorrhage and comparison with computed tomography. Radiology 139:687–691, 1981.

25. Kosmetatos N, Dinter C, Williams ML, Lourie H, Berne AS. Intracranial hemorrhage in the premature. Am J Dis Child 134:855–859, 1980.

26. Korobkin R. The relationship between head circumference and the development of communicating hydrocephalus in infants following intraventricular hemorrhage. Pediatrics 56:74–77, 1975.

27. Volpe JJ, Pasternak JF, Allan WC. Ventricular dilatation preceding rapid head growth following neonatal intracranial hemorrhage. Am J Dis Child 131:1212–1215, 1977.

28. Hill A, Volpe JJ. Normal pressure hydrocephalus in the newborn. Pediatrics 68:623–629, 1981.

29. Fleischer AC, Hutchison AA, Bundy AL, Machin JE, Thieme GA, Stahlman MT, James AE Jr. Serial sonography of posthemorrhagic ventricular dilatation and porencephaly after intracranial hemorrhage in the preterm neonate. AJR 141:451–455, 1983.

30. Volpe JJ. Current concepts in neonatal medicine: Neonatal intraventricular hemorrhage. N Engl J Med 304:886–891, 1981.

31. Shankaran S, Slovis TL, Bedard MP, Poland RL. Sonographic classification of intracranial hemorrhage. A prognostic indicator of mortality, morbidity, and short-term neurologic outcome. J Pediatr 100:469–475, 1982.

32. Allan WC, Holt PJ, Sawyer LR, Tito AM, Meade SK. Ventricular dilation after neonatal periventricular-intraventricular hemorrhage. Am J Dis Child 136:589–593, 1982.

33. Mantovani JF, Pasternak JF, Mathew OP. Failure of daily lumbar punctures to prevent the development of hydrocephalus following intraventricular hemorrhage. J Pediatr 97:278–281, 1980.

34. LeBlanc R, O'Gorman AM. Neonatal intracranial hemorrhage: a clinical and serial computerized tomographic study. J Neurosurg 53:642–651, 1980.

35. Hill A. Ventricular dilatation following intraventricular hemorrhage in the premature infant. Can J Neurol Sci 10:81–85, 1983.

36. Bowerman RA, Donn SM, Silver TM, Jaffe MH. Natural history of neonatal periventricular/intraventricular hemorrhage and its complications: sonographic observations. AJR 143:1041–1052, 1984.

37. Grant EG, Kerner M, Schellinger D, Borts FT, McCullogh DC, Smith Y, Sivasubramanian KN, Davitt MK. Evolution of porencephalic cysts from intraparenchymal hemorrhage in neonates: Sonographic evidence. AJR 138:467–470, 1982.

38. Sauerbrei EE, Digney M, Harrison PB, Cooperberg PL. Ultrasonic evaluation of neonatal intracranial hemorrhage and its complications. Radiology 139:677–685, 1981.

39. Pasternak JF, Mantovani JF, Volpe JJ. Porencephaly from periventricular intracerebral hemorrhage in a premature infant. Am J Dis Child 134:673–675, 1980.

40. Donn SM, Bowerman RA. Neonatal posthemorrhagic porencephaly. Am J Dis Child 136:707–709, 1982.

41. Krishnamoorthy KS, Shannon DC, DeLong GR, Todres ID, Davis KR. Neurologic sequelae in the survivors of neonatal intraventricular hemorrhage. Pediatrics 64:233–237, 1979.

42. Papile L, Munsick-Bruno G, Schaefer A. Relationship of cerebral intraventricular hemorrhage and early childhood neurologic handicaps. J Pediatr 103:273–277, 1983.

43. Banker B, Larroche JC. Periventricular leukomalacia of infancy. Arch Neurol 7:386–409, 1962.

44. Armstrong D, Norman MG. Periventricular leukomalacia: A one-year autopsy study. Arch Dis Child 49:367–375, 1974.

45. Smith YF. Periventricular leukomalacia in the infant and neonate: Incidence and outcome. In this volume: Neurosonography of the Pre-term Neonate. Grant EG, ed. Springer-Verlag, New York, 1986.

46. Grant EG, Schellinger D. Intraventricular hemorrhage and PVL: Sonographic features and clinical outcome. AJNR (in press).

47. Partridge JC, Babcock DS, Steichen JJ, Han BK. Optimal timing for diagnostic cranial ultrasound in low-birth-weight infants: detection of intracranial hemorrhage and ventricular dilation. J Pediatr 102:281–287, 1983.

48. Donn M, Stuck KJ. Neonatal germinal matrix hemorrhage: evidence of a progressive lesion. J Pediatr 99:459–461, 1981.

49. Schellinger D, Grant EG, Richardson JD. Cystic periventricular leukomalacia: sonographic and CT findings. AJNR 5:439–445, 1984.

50. Garrett WJ, Kossoff G, Jones RFC. Ultrasonic cross-sectional visualization of hydrocephalus in infants. Neuroradiology 8:279–288, 1975.

51. Grant EG, Schellinger D, Borts Ft, McCullough DC, Friedman GR, Sivasubramanian KN, Smith Y. Real-time sonography of the neonatal and infant head. AJNR 1:487–492, 1980.

52. Edwards MK, Brown DL, Muller J, Grossman CB, Chua GT. Cribside neurosonography: Real-time sonography for intracranial investigation of the neonate. AJR 136:271–276, 1981.

53. Slovis TL, Kuhns LR. Real-time sonography of

the brain through the anterior fontanelle. AJR 136:277–286, 1981.

54. Ben-Ora A, Eddy L, Hatch G, Solida B. The anterior fontanelle as an acoustic window to the neonatal ventricular system. JCU 8:65–67, 1980.

55. Johnson ML, Mack LA, Rumack CM, Frost M, Rashbaum C. B-Mode echoencephalography in the normal and high-risk infant. AJR 133:375–381, 1979.

56. Babcock DS, Han BK, LeQuesne GW. B-mode gray scale ultrasound of the head in the newborn and young infant. AJR 134:457–468, 1980.

57. Haber K, Wachter RD, Christenson PC, Vaucher Y, Sahn DJ, Smith JR. Ultrasonic evaluation of intracranial pathology in infants: a new technique. Radiology 134:173–178, 1980.

58. Fleischer A, Hutchinson A, Kirchner S, James AE. Cranial sonography of the preterm neonate. Diagn Imaging 3:20–28, 1981.

59. Bowie JD, Kirks DR, Rosenberg ER, Clair MR. Caudothalamic groove: value in identification of germinal matrix hemorrhage by sonography in preterm neonates. AJNR 4:1107–1110, 1983.

60. Hambleton G, Wigglesworth JS. Origin of intraventricular hemorrhage in the preterm neonate. Arch Dis Child 51:651–659, 1976.

61. Larroche JC. Subependymal pseudocyst in the newborn. Biol Neonate 21:170–183, 1972.

62. Larroche JC. Developmental Pathology of the Neonate. Excerpta Medica, Amsterdam, 440–441, 1977.

63. Shackelford GD, Fulling KH, Glasier CM. Cysts of the subependymal germinal matrix: sonographic demonstration with pathologic correlation. Radiology 149:117–121, 1983.

64. Flodmark O, Becker LE, Harwood-Nash DC, Fitzhardinge PM, Fitz CR, Chuang SH. Correlation between computed tomography and autopsy in premature and full-term neonates that have suffered perinatal asphyxia. Radiology 137:93–103, 1980.

65. Friede R. Developmental Neuropathology. Springer-Verlag, New York, 1975.

66. Donat JF, Okasaki H, Kleinberg F, Reagan TJ. Intraventricular hemorrhages in full-term and premature infants. Mayo Clin Proc 53:437–441, 1978.

67. Reeder JD, Kaude JV, Setzer ES. Choroid plexus hemorrhage in premature neonates. AJNR 3:619–622, 1982.

68. Craig WS. Intracranial haemorrhage in the newborn. Arch Dis Child 13:89–124, 1938.

69. Hemsath FA. Ventricular cerebral hemorrhage in the newborn infant. Am J Obstet Gynecol 26:343–354, 1934.

70. Dunnick NR, Schuette W, Shawker T. Ultrasonic demonstration of thrombus in the common carotid artery. AJR 133:544–545, 1979.

71. Mittelstaedt C, Volberg F, Merten D, Brill PW. The sonographic diagnosis of neonatal adrenal hemorrhage. Radiology 131:453–457, 1979.

72. Demaria A, Bommer W, Neumann A, et al. Left ventricular thrombi identified by cross-sectional echocardiography. Ann Intern Med 90:14–18, 1979.

73. Brown R. Ultrasonography: Basic Principles and Clinical Applications. Warren H. Green, St. Louis, 1975.

74. Goss SA, Johnston R, Dunn F. Comprehensive compilation of empirical ultrasound property of mammalian tissues. J Acoust Soc Am 64:423–457, 1978.

75. Zana R, Lang J. Interaction of ultrasound and amniotic liquid. Ultrasound Med Biol 1:253–254, 1974.

76. Wladimiroff J, Craft I, Talbert D. In vitro measurements of sound velocity in human fetal brain tissue. Ultrasound Med biol 1:377–382, 1975.

77. Bradley E, Sacario J. The velocity of ultrasound in human blood under varying physiologic parameters. J Surg Res 12:290–297, 1972.

78. Bakke T, Gytre T, Haagensen A, and Giezendanner L. Ultrasonic measurement of sound velocity in whole blood. Scand J Clin Lab Invest 35:473–478, 1975.

79. Larroche JC. Post-haemorrhagic hydrocephalus in infancy: anatomical study. Biol Neonate 20:287–299, 1972.

80. Mack LA, Wright K, Hirsch JH, Alvord EC, Guthrie RD, Shuman WP, Rogers JV, and Bolender NF. Intracranial hemorrhage in premature infants: accuracy of sonographic evaluation. AJR 137:245–250, 1982.

81. Fiske CE, Filly RA, Callen PW. The normal choroid plexus: ultrasonographic appearance of the neonatal head. Radiology 141:467–471, 1981.

82. Netanyahu I, Grant EG. Sonography of the choroid plexus in infants with spinal dysraphism: normal variant versus intraventricular hematoma. AJNR 7:317–321, 1986.

83. Silverboard G, Horder MH, Ahmann PA, Schwartz JF. Reliability of ultrasound in diagnosis of intracerebral hemorrhage and posthemorrhagic hydrocephalus: comparison with computed tomography. Pediatrics 66:507–514, 1980.

84. Wicks JD, Silver TM, Bree RL. Gray-scale features of hematomas, ultrasonic spectrum. AJR 131:977–980, 1978.

85. Fawer CL, Levene M. Elusive blood clots and

fluctuating ventricular dilatation after neonatal intraventricular haemorrhage. Arch Dis Child 57:158–160, 1982.

86. Kibler RF, Couch RSC, Crompton MR. Hydrocephalus in the adult following spontaneous subarachnoid hemorrhage. Brain 84:45–61, 1961.

87. Grant EG, Schellinger DS, Richardson JD. Real-time ultrasonography of the posterior fossa. J Ultrasound Med 2:73–87, 1983.

88. Grant EG. Update on neurosonography. In: Ultrasound Annual 1984. Sanders RC, Hill M, eds. Raven, New York, 161–210, 1984.

89. Taylor GA, Sanders RC. Dandy–Walker syndrome: recognition by sonography. AJNR 4:1203–1206, 1983.

90. Kim MS, Elyaderani MK. Sonographic diagnosis of cerebroventricular hemorrhage in utero. Radiology 142:479–480, 1982.

91. Chinn DH, Filly RA. Extensive intracranial hemorrhage in utero. J Ultrasound Med 2:285–287, 1983.

92. Donn SM, DiPietro MA, Faix RG, Bowerman RA. The sonographic appearance of old intraventricular hemorrhage present at birth. J Ultrasound Med 2:283–284, 1983.

93. McGahan JP, Haesslein HC, Meyers M, Ford KB. Sonographic recognition of in utero intraventricular hemorrhage. AJR 142:171–173, 1984.

94. Molteni RA, Gammon K, D'Souza BJ, Altman J, Freeman JM, Shinnar S. Intraventricular hemorrhage in the premature infant: a changing outlook. N Engl J Med 306:1464–1468, 1982.

95. Levene MI, Starte DR. A longitudinal study of posthaemorrhagic ventricular dilatation in the newborn. Arch Dis Child 56:905–910, 1981.

96. Allan WC, Holt PJ, Sawyer LR, Tito AM, Kellogg MS. Ventricular dilatation after neonatal periventricular-intraventricular hemorrhage. Am J Dis Child 136:589–594, 1982.

97. Graziani L, Dave R, Desai H, Branca P, Waldroup L. Ultrasound studies in preterm infants with hydrocephalus. Pediatrics 97:624–630, 1980.

98. Bada HS, Salmon JH, Pearson DH. Early surgical intervention in post-haemorrhagic hydrocephalus. Childs Brain 5:109–115, 1979.

99. De SN. A study of the changes in the brain in experimental internal hydrocephalus. J Pathol 62:197–208, 1950.

100. Weller RO, Wisniewski H, Shulman K, Terry RD. Experimental hydrocephalus in young dogs: histological and ultrastructural study of the brain tissue damage. J Neuropathol Exp Neurol 30:613–626, 1971.

101. Rowlatt U. The microscopic effects of ventricular dilatation without increase in head size. J Neurosurg 48:957–961, 1978.

102. Johnson MA, Pennock JM, Bydder GM, Steiner RE, Thomas DJ, Hayward R, Bryant DR, Payne JA, Levine MI, Whitelaw A, et al. Clinical NMR imaging of the brain in children: normal and neurological disease. AJR 141:1005–1018, 1983.

103. Papile LA, Burstein J, Burstein R, Koffler H, Koops BL, Johnson JD. Posthemorrhagic hydrocephalus in low-birth-weight infants: treatment by serial lumbar punctures. J Pediatr 97:273–277, 1980.

104. Mantovani JF, Pasternak JF, Mathew OP, Allan WC, Mills MT, Casper J, Volpe JJ. Failure of daily lumbar punctures to prevent the development of hydrocephalus following intraventricular hemorrhage. J Pediatr 97:278–281, 1980.

105. Fiske CE, Filly RA, Callen PW. Sonographic measurement of lateral ventricular width in early ventricular dilation. JCU 9:303–307, 1981.

106. Levene MI. Measurement of the growth of the lateral ventricles in preterm infants with real-time ultrasound. Arch Dis Child 56:900–904, 1981.

107. Grant EG, Borts F, Schellinger D, McCullough DC, Smith Y. Cerebral intraparenchymal hemorrhage in the neonate: sonographic appearance. AJNR 2:129–132, 1981.

108. Horbar JD, Pasnick M, Lucey JF. Ultrasound detection of cerebral cavitation following needle puncture of the lateral ventricles. JCU 10:406–408, 1982.

109. Lyon G, Robain O. Etude comparative des encephalopathies circulatories prenatales et paranatales (hydranencephalies, porencephalies et encephalomalacias kystiques de la substance blanche). Acta Neuropathol (Berl) 9:79–98, 1967.

110. Stevenson LD, McGowan LE. Encephalomalacia with cavity formation in infants. Arch Pathol Lab Med 34:286–330, 1942.

111. Friede RL. Developmental Neuropathology. New York, Springer-Verlag, 1975.

112. Grunnet ML, Shields WD. Cerebellar hemorrhage in the premature infant. J Pediatr 88:605–608, 1976.

113. Martin R. Roessmann U, Fanaroff A. Massive intracerebellar hemorrhage in low birthweight infants. J Pediatr 89:290–293, 1976.

114. Pape KE, Armstrong DL, Fitzhardinge PM. Central nervous system pathology associated with mask ventilation in the very low birth weight infant: a new etiology for intracerebellar hemorrhages. Pediatrics 58:473–483, 1976.

115. Shuman RM, Oliver TK. Face masks defended. Pediatrics 58:621–623, 1976.
116. Foy P, Dubbins PA, Waldroup L, Grazianik L, Goldberg BB, Berry R. Ultrasound demonstration of cerebellar hemorrhage in a neonate. JCU 10:196–198, 1982.
117. Reeder JD, Setzer ES, Kaude JV. Ultrasonographic detection of perinatal intracerebellar hemorrhage. Pediatrics 70:385–386, 1982.
118. Perlman JM, Nelson JS, McAlister WH, Volpe JJ. Intracerebellar hemorrhage in a premature newborn: diagnosis by real-time ultrasound and correlation with autopsy findings. Pediatrics 71:159–162, 1983.
119. Peterson CM, Smith WL, Franken EA. Neonatal intracerebellar hemorrhage: detection by real-time ultrasound. Radiology 150:391–392, 1984.
120. Scotti G, Flodmark O, Harwood-Nash DC, Humphries RP. Posterior fossa hemorrhages in the newborn. Comput Assist Tomogr 5:68–72, 1981.
121. Fishman MA, Percy AK, Cheek WR, Speer ME. Successful conservative management of cerebellar hematomas in term neonates. J Pediatr 98:466–468, 1981.

4
Neurosonography: Periventricular Leukomalacia

Edward G. Grant

There are references to periventricular leuko-malacia (PVL) in the medical literature dating as far back as 1843,[1] when Little delivered a series of lectures drawing attention to the association of spasmodic contractures and mental retardation with prematurity. Although Virchow[2] and Parrot[3-5] described the pathology and resultant clinical abnormalities of PVL in remarkable detail, few additional reports of PVL appeared in the literature until Banker and Larroche investigated it in 1962.[6] Their classic work did much to elucidate the incidence, predisposing factors, clinical features, and pathology of PVL.

Banker and Larroche described PVL as "the most common pathologic change in the brain of newborn infants." In addition, they found that patients affected by this infarctive process invariably exhibited profound clinical deficits, prominent among which were the spastic diplegia and quadriplegia alluded to by Little over 100 years before. The high frequency and devastating nature of PVL should have spurred intensive investigation into this subject, but once again, few investigators took up the cause. Radiographically, PVL was not even described until 1978, when Di Chiro et al. reported the computed tomography (CT) findings in four cases.[7]

The discovery of the high incidence of germinal matrix-related hemorrhage (GMRH) in the preterm neonate pushed PVL far into the background in the latter half of the 1970s. Neonatal neuroinvestigation became almost exclusively focused on intracranial hemorrhage. In 1982–1983, however, three separate groups described a "new" abnormality in the brain of the pre-term neonate.[8-10] This new abnormality was PVL. The pathologic findings were the same as had been described a century before—softening and eventual cystic necrosis of the periventricular white matter. The circumstances under which PVL occurred and was diagnosed, however, were completely different. Today, in the setting of the intensive care nursery, PVL constitutes a unique disease process that affects a specific population and can be followed sonographically from its inception through its various phases.

A number of authors[6, 11-13] have contributed to the understanding of the pathologic evolution of PVL over the years, and knowledge of the pathology definitely enhances one's ability to understand its sonography. Following the initial infarction, coagulation necrosis occurs. Armstrong and Norman[12] demonstrated hemorrhage into the infarction in 7 of their 28 patients. The areas of infarction/hemorrhage undergo cystic degeneration, which results in periventricular cysts. These cysts may vary in size from a few millimeters to extensive zones of breakdown that communicate freely with the ventricles. Both De Reuck et al[11] and Armstrong and Norman[12] found gliosis and scarring eventually replaced the periventricular cysts in many cases. This scarring left little evidence of the original insult on gross examination of older autopsy specimens with the exception of unusual, localized forms of ventriculomegaly. Other late findings in PVL include generalized cerebral wasting typified by ex vacuuo ventricular enlargement, widening of the cerebral sulci, and overall decrease in brain mass.[7, 11]

Along the lines of the evolving pathology of

PVL, we can define two specific sonographic phases of the disease. The first of these is the acute or echogenic phase, the sonographic expression of the initial infarction and/or hemorrhage. These areas of increased echogenicity eventually undergo liquefaction necrosis, leading to what we have termed cystic PVL.[14] As the immediate periventricular insult evolves from its acute to chronic form, other more peripheral or global effects from the initial insult may also become evident, and these are discussed separately.

Sonographic Diagnosis of PVL

The classic or full-blown sonographic picture of the acute phase of PVL is quite striking. It consists of broad bands of markedly increased echogenicity surrounding both lateral ventricles. This may be easily identified from any scan plane, either semiaxial or parasagittal (Fig. 4-1 A and B). In severe cases, as illustrated, this increased echogenicity extends from the anterior to the posterior periventricular white matter and even extends toward the temporal horns. The abnormally increased periventricular echogenicity is isoechoic with the choroid plexus. In most cases, a small quantity of hematoma will be present within the ventricles. This hematoma is as reflective as the choroid plexus medially and the PVL laterally, resulting in two large continuous echo complexes. Because this process is usually symmetric, one periventricular area is the mirror image of the other. PVL may occasionally be unilateral (Fig. 4-2), although we have found this unusual, particularly during the echogenic phase.

In some patients, foci of higher or lower level echogenicity will be scattered within the general halo of increased echogenicity about the lateral ventricles (Fig. 4-3, A and B). These foci of particularly high reflectivity may be caused by a thick hemorrhagic infarct. The intensely echogenic areas could also represent the most severely involved portions of the brain, the actual watershed zones between the cerebral arteries.

The echogenic phase of PVL is usually quite obvious at sonography; however, two major factors complicate its diagnosis. The first and most important factor is the existence of a nor-

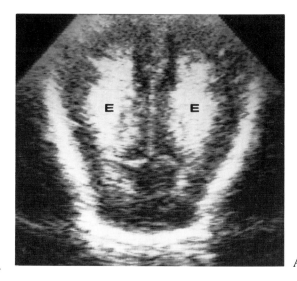

A

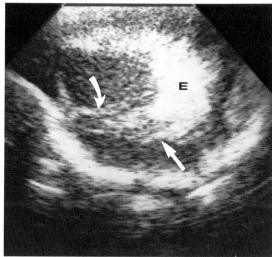

B

FIGURE 4-1. Angled coronal (**A**) and parasagittal (**B**) sections in 3-day-old neonate with bilateral PVL. Intensely echogenic areas (*E*) surround both lateral ventricles. Internal echogenicity is homogeneous, continuous, and isoechoic with choroid plexus. **A**, On coronal section, one zone of PVL is the mirror image of the opposite. **B**, On parasagittal section (**B**), abnormal echogenicity extends inferiorly to almost surround temporal horn (*straight arrow*) below Sylvian fissure (*curved arrow*).

mal band of increased echogenicity around the ventricles (Fig. 4-4 A and B). The actual etiology of these bands remains uncertain; we have postulated that they may represent a scanning artifact because they are not easily reproduced from all scanning planes. Periventricular echogenicity, however, could be increased by the

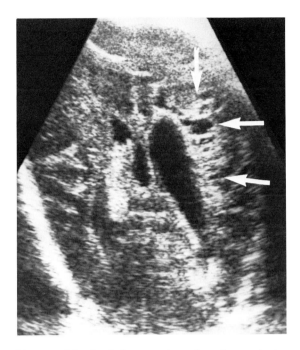

FIGURE 4-2. Angled coronal section demonstrates periventricular cysts and abnormal areas of increased echogenicity about left lateral ventricle (*arrows*). These findings are typical of cystic PVL, but unusual because they are unilateral.

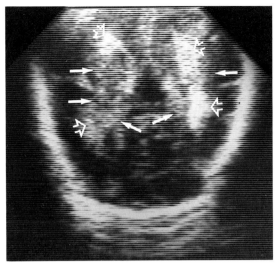

A

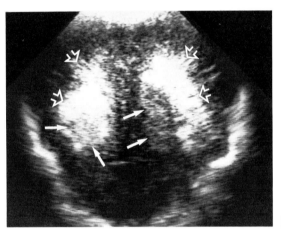

B

FIGURE 4-3. Angled coronal sections in two neonates with bilateral PVL. **A**, Scattered foci of intense echogenicity (*open arrows*) within generally increased periventricular echogenicity (*arrows*). **B**, In this child, higher echogenicity (*open arrows*) predominates over areas of lesser echogenicity (*arrows*).

numerous interfaces provided by the abundant venous channels that exist around the lateral ventricles. We have termed this normal finding "the periventricular echogenic halo."[10] While this normal echo halo may mimic PVL in some patients, a number of sonographic observations can be useful in differentiating between the two. The most important of these differentiating factors is the ease of reproducing true PVL in any scanning plane. The normal periventricular halo is not easily reproducible from all angles. Normal periventricular echogenicity seen in the semiaxial planes (Fig. 4-4 A) is not reproduced when one scans lateral to the ventricles in a parasagittal orientation. Similarly, one cannot identify the normally increased echogenicity seen in the area of the posterior striations on parasagittal sections when scanning superior to the ventricles in the semiaxial plane (Fig. 4-4 B). True PVL should even be evident when scanning through the skull (Fig. 4-5).

Other methods of differentiating between the normal echo halo and PVL exist. Normal periventricular echogenicity should never be as intense as the echogenicity seen with PVL. Therefore, the normal echo halo should be less reflective than the choroid plexus. In normal patients, a thin line of anechoic cerebrospinal fluid (CSF) should also separate the normal echo halo from the choroid plexus. Because at least a small amount of intraventricular hemorrhage (IVH) almost always accompanies PVL, this line of demarcation should be lost. One should find a large, continuous echo complex consisting of choroid plexus, PVL, and IVH. This is well demonstrated in Fig. 4-1. PVL may

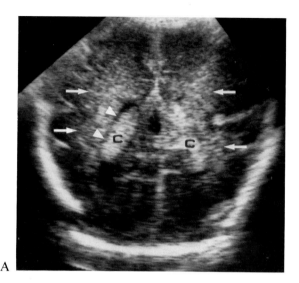

A

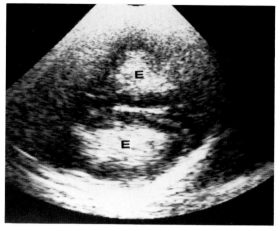

FIGURE 4-5. Transcranial sonogram in child with PVL. Large abnormally echogenic areas (*E*) are clearly visible around both lateral ventricles even when scanning through temporal squamosa.

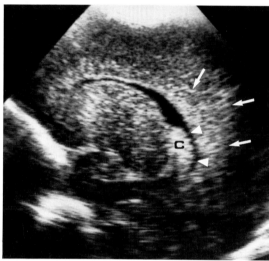

B

FIGURE 4-4. Semiaxial (**A**) and parasagittal (**B**) sections showing normal periventricular echogenic halo. Areas of relatively high-level echogenicity (*arrows*) parallel both lateral ventricles in semiaxial orientation and are located superior to the ventricular trigone in the parasagittal plane. Normal periventricular echogenicity tends to be internally homogeneous and have irregular, poorly defined borders. The normal echogenic halo should be less echogenic than the choroid plexus (*C*) and separated from it by a thin line of anechoic CSF (*arrowheads*).

also be diagnosed by identifying areas of inhomogeneity in the echo halo, as illustrated in Figs. 4-3 A and B. The normal echo halo should be relatively homogeneous, whereas PVL may contain scattered blotchy areas of very high-level echogenicity. The borders of the

normal periventricular echogenicity should also gradually blend into the surrounding cerebral echogenicity. This is not the case in PVL; its borders are well defined and end abruptly, although they are typically quite ragged.

Familiarity with the scanning characteristics of one particular machine or one frequency transducer is also important in differentiating PVL from the normal echo halo. Image contrast characteristics may vary from one piece of ultrasound equipment to the next, and confusion about normal versus abnormal periventricular echogenicity may arise on this basis (Fig. 4-6 A and B). One must become accustomed to the normal appearance of periventricular echogenicity produced by any one scanner; abnormal echogenicity will then be more apparent. Similarly, variations in system gain, in film contrast, and in developing technique can also confuse the issue. These latter three problems, however, can only occur if the physician is not present when the actual scan is performed.

The differentiation between the normal echo halo and PVL may occasionally be impossible. In a small minority of children, the answer may remain unclear over a number of successive scans. In these cases, late follow-up may provide the only real answer by identifying periventricular cysts, thereby confirming PVL. Whether or not any reason exists for the particularly high-level periventricular echogenicity

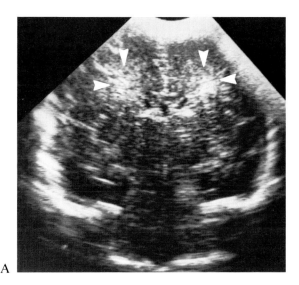

A

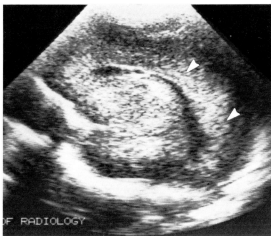

B

FIGURE 4-6. Normal semiaxial (**A**) and parasagittal (**B**) scans that mimic PVL. Incorrectly adjusted contrast may render periventricular echoes (*arrowheads*) artifactually prominent. Periventricular echogenicity frequently appears particularly bright in comparison to surrounding cerebral parenchyma when scanning with the 7.5-MHz transducer. In certain patients, differentiation between high-level yet apparently normal periventricular echogenicity and PVL may be impossible; follow-up scans eventually yield a definite answer when cysts become evident or fail to appear.

seen in some neonates remains uncertain. One could even postulate that these children with transient, high-level periventricular echogenicity may be manifesting cerebral infarction that never undergoes cystic degeneration, merely gliosis and scarring.

A second source of confusion in the diagnosis of PVL lies in its differentiation from intraparenchymal hemorrhage (IPH) (Grade IV cerebroventricular hemorrhage). While PVL in its full bilateral form should never be confused with IPH, the more focal forms of PVL may be identical. These focal forms of PVL are typically located in two areas, anteriorly, lateral to the frontal horn in the centrum semiovale of Yakolev and/or the corona radiata (Fig. 4-7 A), and posteriorly, atop the ventricular trigone (Fig. 4-7 B) in the region of the posterior striations. Shuman and Selednick found this posterior infarction zone to be the area most frequently affected in PVL.[13]

In attempting to distinguish between focal PVL and IPH, it must be remembered that IPH may extend far into the periphery of the brain, seemingly almost to the dura. PVL, on the other hand, is always limited to the region immediately about the ventricles. Additionally, copious amounts of IVH are usually associated with IPH; a paucity of hematoma in the lateral ventricles is more typical of PVL. PVL most frequently involves the area above the lateral ventricular trigones; IPH may dissect toward that region, but should not actually be in contact with the ventricular wall (Fig. 4-8 B). Focal PVL in the anterior watershed zone is most difficult to differentiate from IPH. IPH is always most pronounced anteriorly near the germinal matrix, and frequently limited to that area. The two may actually be impossible to differentiate sonographically. In the coronal plane, IPH should typically be broad based against the ventricle, whereas PVL most often has a thinner waist centrally and gradually increases in width peripherally (Fig. 4-8 A).

We have stressed that minimal IVH is typical of PVL (Fig. 4-9). Significant IVH, however, has occurred in association with PVL in approximately 25% of our patients (Fig. 4-10, A–E). It is of yet unknown if these two processes are actually related. In some cases the IVH may represent centripetal extension from hemorrhagic PVL. In others, IVH may originate in the germinal matrix. PVL and IVH in the same patient are also not necessarily temporally related. We have seen cases where the two occurred at different times. We further postulate that one infant had PVL, IVH, and IPH. This neonate had bilateral PVL identified on the

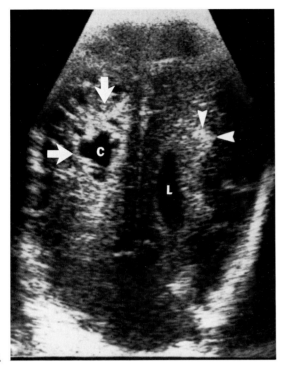

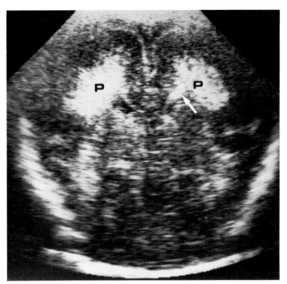

A

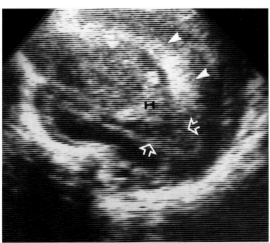

B

FIGURE 4-7. Focal PVL. **A**, Semiaxial section shows isolated area of increased echogenicity (*arrowheads*) about left lateral ventricle (*L*). Note more extensive PVL on right (*arrows*) that has already begun to undergo cystic necrosis (*C*). **B**, Parasagittal section reveals isolated PVL (*arrowheads*) in area of posterior striations above ventricular trigone. Posterior ventricle (*open arrows*) is mildly enlarged and contains small amount of hematoma (*H*). (From Grant EG, Schellinger D, 1985.[16])

FIGURE 4-8. PVL versus IPH. **A**, Semiaxial section shows bilateral PVL in anterior watershed zones (*P*). IPH should be broad based against lateral ventricle. PVL has narrow waist (*arrow*) and spreads out peripherally. **B**, Parasagittal section shows dissection of IPH (*I*) posteriorly from region of germinal matrix hemorrhage (*G*). Note large intraventricular hematoma (*H*). Parenchymal hematoma is separated from ventricle by a zone of normal tissue (*arrowhead*) but is continuous with germinal matrix hemorrhage (*arrow*).

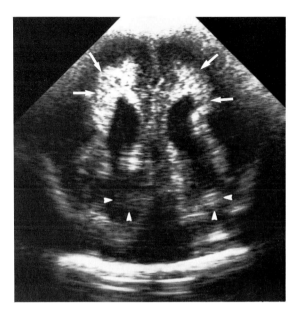

FIGURE 4-9. Semiaxial section from 2-week-old child with bilateral PVL (*arrows*) and mild ventriculomegaly. Note small amount of intraventricular hematoma (*arrowheads*) shown to good advantage because of surrounding CSF. Early on, small amounts of IVH may be difficult to see because it is isoechoic with choroid plexus and PVL.

first examination at 1 day of age. A follow-up scan at day four, after a catastrophic clinical event, revealed a huge right-sided area of what appeared to be IPH in addition to the PVL seen earlier (Figs. 4-11 A and B). The forces at work behind PVL, germinal matrix hemorrhage (GMH), and IPH in the same patient are poorly understood; the actual relationship, if any, between these entities remains to be further investigated. Regardless of the temporal or even the etiologic relationship that may or may not exist between PVL and IVH, their occurrence in the same patient has resulted in extremely difficult neurosurgical management in the majority of our cases. These children have particularly poor prognoses.[15]

The cystic or more chronic phase of PVL is, in many ways, the true sonographic hallmark of the entire process; diagnosing the acute or echogenic phase may at times be quite confusing. Levene[10] has reported cases in which cystic PVL was the only sonographic manifestation of the process. Schellinger,[15] however, in a review of a large number of cases, contended that periventricular echogenicity is always abnormally increased to some degree early in the course of PVL. As the sonologist involved in making these diagnoses, I must admit that the prospective identification of the more subtle cases of PVL may be quite difficult if not occasionally impossible on the basis of increased echogenicity alone. Certainly, the sonologist must equivocate in a small number of cases, lest he unduly alarm the neonatologist by making too many falsely positive diagnoses. In cystic PVL, on the other hand, the sonographic findings should be unequivocal.

Cystic PVL usually first appears within the existing abnormal periventricular echogenicity. In some cases, it however, may appear de novo. The time when these cystic areas are first visible is quite variable. They may appear as early as 10 days after the initial insult, or as late as 20. We have examined one neonate who had cystic PVL on the first day of life, implying that the initial insult occurred in utero.

Early on, periventricular cysts may be quite small and scattered within the abnormally echogenic areas around the lateral ventricles. These small cysts may only be visible using the high-resolution scanner (Fig. 4-12 A and B). Eventually the cysts enlarge or coalesce as the echogenic infarction liquifies further. In localized or less severe cases of PVL, cysts may be limited to the areas of the corona radiata anteriorly (Fig. 4-13 A), or to the area superior to the ventricular trigones posteriorly (Fig. 4-13 B). These two areas correspond to the circulatory watershed zones described earlier. More frequently, extensive areas of cystic degeneration parallel the bodies of the lateral ventricles. Cysts may extend from almost the tip of the frontal horn to well posterior to the occipital horn. The extent of the cystic degeneration usually closely approximates the extent of the original echogenic infarction unless posthemorrhagic hydrocephalus complicates the situation. Cystic PVL is usually best demonstrated lateral to the ventricles in the semiaxial orientation and somewhat superior to the ventricles in the parasagittal plane (Fig. 4-14 A and B).

Cystic PVL may only manifest itself by the formation of very small cysts. Pathologically, cysts of 2–3 mm may be the only gross find-

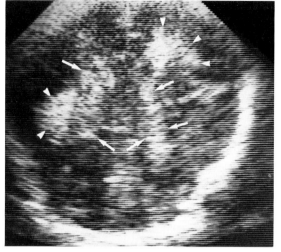

FIGURE 4-10. Semiaxial (**A**) and right (**B**) and left (**C**) parasagittal sections taken at 1 week. Scattered areas of abnormal intraparenchymal echogenicity typical of PVL are noted about both lateral ventricles (*arrowheads*). A large amount of intraventricular hematoma is also present (*arrows*). Right and left parasagittal sections (**D** and **E**) from follow-up scan at 6 weeks show marked enlargement of both lateral ventricles (*L*) and extensive areas of cystic degeneration (*C*). Ventricular shunt was eventually placed and required multiple revisions.

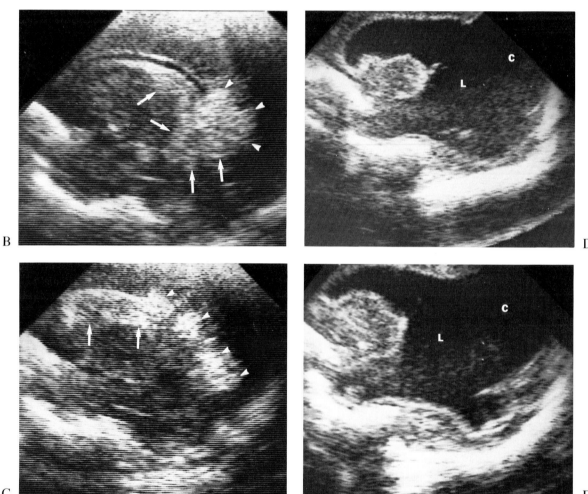

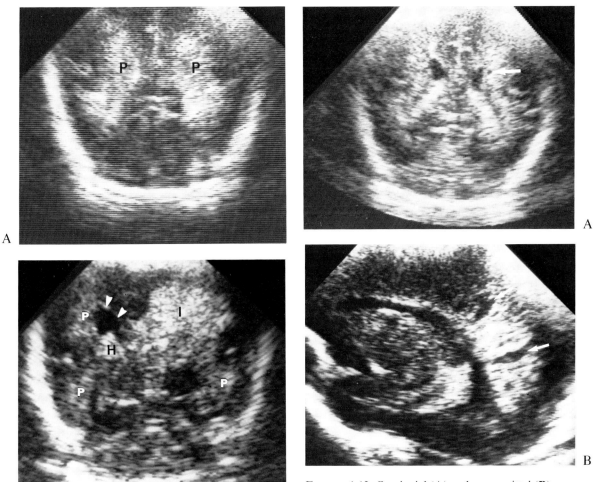

B

FIGURE 4-11. PVL and IPH in same patient. **A**, 1-day-old neonate with bilateral PVL (*P*). **B**, Same patient at 4 days of age now shows large left IPH (*I*) and persistence of abnormal periventricular echogenicity (*P*). Note interval appearance of IVH (*H*) and ventriculomegaly (*arrowheads*). This child also required ventricular shunting and multiple revisions.

FIGURE 4-12. Semiaxial (**A**) and parasagittal (**B**) sections reveal small cystic areas (*arrows*) within echogenic zones of PVL. These are the first manifestations of liquefaction of periventricular infarction.

ing.[7, 11, 13] A review of our own cases shows that a significant percentage of cases of PVL may go unnoticed by using only the routine 5 MHz scanner.[16] Since cystic PVL may be the only certain manifestation of the disease, the identification of cysts as small as possible is imperative (Fig. 4-15 A and B).

In severe cases, cystic PVL may be extensive enough to mimic generalized ventricular enlargement (Fig. 4-16 A and B). Although these areas of cystic necrosis may be larger than the

ventricles themselves, the presence of internal septations usually betrays their origin. Such septations are best seen in less complicated cases of PVL such as are illustrated in Figs. 4-14, A and B. The septations probably represent residual fibrous stromal elements of the brain that were not destroyed by the infarction. Curiously, these septae are seldom seen following IPH; they are either totally destroyed or pushed aside by the hematoma, resulting in a focal unilocular porencephalic cyst. The septations typical of cystic PVL frequently break down over time. In many cases, even the ependyma separating the ventricle from the cysts will degenerate, leaving a large defect in apparent open

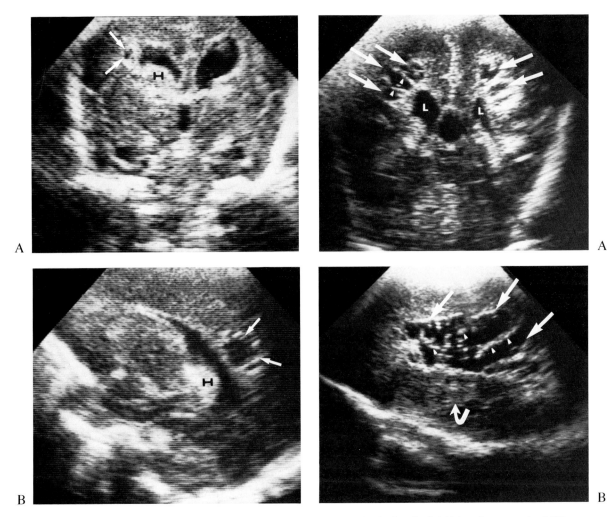

FIGURE 4-13. Coronal section (**A**) from 3-week-old infant reveals small focus of cystic PVL (*arrows*) in area of right corona radiata. Parasagittal section (**B**) in 4-week-old infant shows localized region of cystic PVL in area of the posterior striations (*arrows*). Note intraventricular hematoma (*H*) and ventriculomegaly in both sections.

FIGURE 4-14. Semiaxial (**A**) and parasagittal (**B**) sections in infants with typical findings of cystic PVL. Multiple cysts (*arrows*) parallel lateral ventricles. Increased echogenicity continues to surround left lateral ventricle in **A**. Note prominent "septations" in both cases (*arrowheads*). Lateral ventricles (*L*) are of relatively normal size in **A**. Because PVL is located lateral to ventricles in parasagittal plane, they are not visible in **B**. Peripheral location of cysts is indicated by presence of Sylvian fissure (*curved arrow*) in same section (**B**).

communication with the lateral ventricle. Extensive areas of cystic PVL are particularly prominent in children with a combination of PVL and IVH.[15]

Whether PHH plays a role in further complicating PVL is not certain. Surely, communication between an obstructed ventricle and a periventricular cyst could cause the cyst to enlarge. From the sonographic standpoint, one may be unable to clearly differentiate between what is enlarged ventricle and what is cyst. These extensive areas of cystic degeneration may blend imperceptively into the ventricle, creating what we have termed "pseudoventricles." Cystic PVL may only appear as an unusual bulge or irregularity in the contour of the apparent ventricular wall. In a number of cases, only the very anterior portion of the lateral ventricle could be identified (Fig. 4-17 A). In one infant a particularly echogenic "septum"

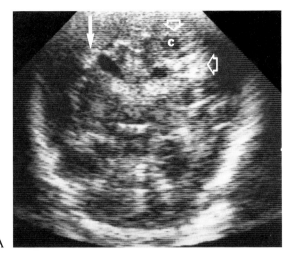

A

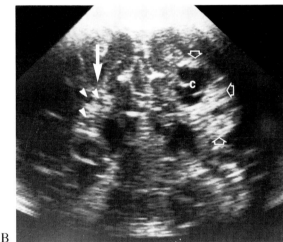

B

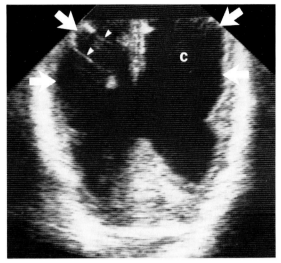

A

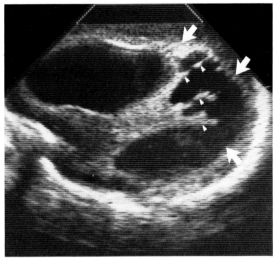

B

FIGURE 4-15. Semiaxial sections taken using 5.0-MHz (**A**) 7.5-MHz (**B**) transducer. Both scans show evidence of cystic (*C*) and echogenic (*open arrows*) PVL on left. Suggestion of increased echogenicity is present on right (*arrow*) using 5.0-MHz technique. Higher resolution scan clearly identifies small cysts (*arrowheads*) within right-sided echogenicity.

FIGURE 4-16. Semiaxial (**A**) and right parasagittal (**B**) sections reveal extensive areas of periventricular cystic degeneration or formation of "pseudoventricles" (*arrows*). Septations (*arrowheads*) and review of previous scans showing echogenic PVL betray ischemic origins of these areas. It is impossible to tell where true ventricular enlargement ends and "pseudoventricles" begin. These scans are the 8-week follow-up of the neonate with both PVL and IPH shown in Fig. 4-11 A and B. Note that cystic area on left (*C*) corresponds to previous large IPH; it contains no septations.

hinted at the demarcation between ventricle and cyst (Fig. 4-17 B). This "septum" actually represented the remaining portion of the ependyma of the roof of the frontal horn. Identification of some portion of the ventricle is important in these children, as surgical intervention can only effectively decrease the size of the lateral ventricles; minimal decrease in the size of the periventricular cysts can be expected. This phenomenon is quite similar to what occurs in severe cases of IPH. Both are probably the

result of extensive destruction of cerebral tissue.

In patients with localized areas of ventricular enlargement and no prior sonograms to establish the etiology, one may diagnose PVL by

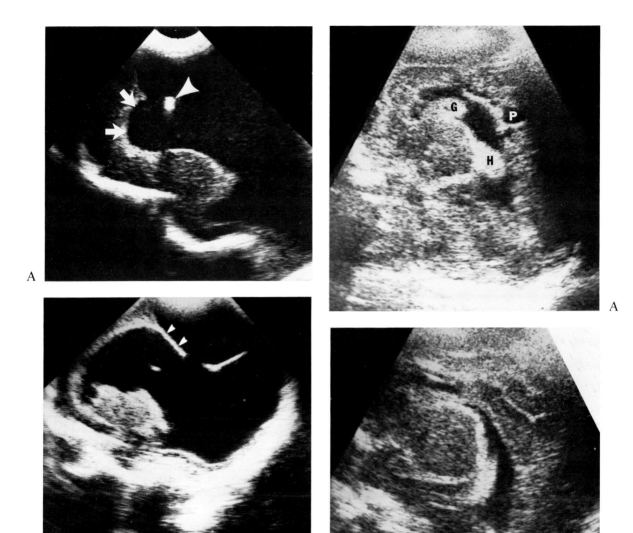

FIGURE 4-17. Parasagittal sections from two infants with "pseudoventricles." **A**, Only anterior tip of frontal horn (*arrows*) is preserved. Remaining portion of ependyma appears as isolated septum (*arrowheads*) in **B**. Shunt (*arrowhead*) has been inserted in **A**, but ventricle has not significantly decreased in size.

FIGURE 4-18. **A**, Parasagittal sections through left lateral ventricle reveals small area of isolated cystic PVL posteriorly (*P*) that is not identified in scan (**B**) performed 3 months later. Note decrease in overall size of lateral ventricle and resorption of both intraventricular hematoma (*H*) and germinal matrix hemorrhage (*G*).

identifying fine septae. CT does not optimally identify these thin membranes, because they are frequently averaged out of the image. Schellinger[14] points out that patients with localized "pseudoventricles" secondary to PVL will often have a persistent scalloped edge to the apparent ventricle even after the septae have broken down. This may be the only finding that differentiates true ventricular enlargement from pseudoventricular enlargement secondary to PVL. This may be further complicated because both "pseudoventricles" may have a similar appearance. The reason for differentiating between actual ventricular enlargement and

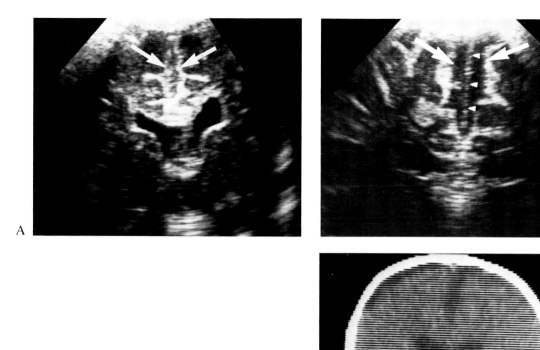

FIGURE 4-19. Coronal (**A**) and axial (**B**) sections showing atrophy. Interhemispheric fissure is widened (*arrows*), and falx (*arrowheads*) is visible as a separate structure in **B**. **C**, Note similar findings on CT scan but superior demonstration of full extent of atrophic process.

pseudoventricles obviously lies in effectiveness of treatment. One may decrease real ventriculomegaly with a shunt, but until the surgeon can replace brain parenchyma, the PVL and its associated neurologic deficits will remain.

Approximately 25% of our children with PVL have had significant IVH and require close follow-up. The remaining 75%, however, do not have significant IVH, major ventricular enlargement, or any other complication requiring treatment. Patients with uncomplicated PVL, therefore, require few scans once associated IVH has been ruled out. In these uncomplicated cases, the periventricular cysts remain relatively static in size. In some, the septae may degenerate over time, leading to moderate cases of pseudoventriculomegaly, but again these require no treatment. In others, all sonographic evidence of PVL may disappear over time. We have followed a number of cases in which small periventricular cysts resolved and the scans returned to normal (Fig. 4-18 A and B). The normal sonogram in such a situation does not change the diagnosis. The pathology of

PVL explains why: The cysts may indeed resolve. Microscopic evaluation, however, shows that the cysts are actually obliterated by gliosis or scarring; the original diagnosis and its associated deficits remain.[11, 12]

The sonographic abnormalities that we have described thus far in PVL are the localized effects of periventricular infarction. Other less focal cerebral abnormalities also occur in a high percentage of these patients. Among our population, findings of generalized atrophy have been typical of the overall picture of PVL.[16] Similar findings of global cerebral wasting were common in the autopsy studies of DeReuck et al.[11] and Shuman and Selednick.[13] One could easily postulate why PVL patients should have diffuse cerebral wasting. The central loss of cerebral tissue alone might account for decreased brain mass in PVL. Another possible etiology could be generalized anoxia. If severe enough, it may cause localized infarction, which is clearly evident early on as PVL. At the same time, however, it may effect the entire brain. The usual effect of global cerebral oxygen deprivation is generalized cerebral wasting or cerebral atrophy.[17]

The sonographic features of cerebral atrophy are the same whether or not they are associated with PVL. Babcock and Ball have described the findings in term neonates with postasphyxial atrophy[17]; our findings in preterm infants with PVL and cerebral atrophy are similar.[16] We have discovered that a very high percentage of neonates with PVL have atrophy. At sonography, the sine qua non of cerebral atrophy is widening of the interhemispheric fissure (Fig. 4-19 A). The cerebral hemispheres are separated by anechoic CSF. Using high-resolution equipment, one may actually demonstrate the surface of the brain, because it is separated from the transducer by the enlarged subarachnoid space. The falx frequently also becomes visible as a separate structure because it is surrounded by fluid (Fig. 4-19 B). These findings about the interhemispheric fissure are often representative of the widened state of all the cerebral sulci, but most are covered by bone and therefore not visible to the sonographer. Comparison of the sonographic findings with a CT scan, however, illustrates that the widened interhemispheric truly does reflect the state of the entire brain surface (Fig. 4-19 C).

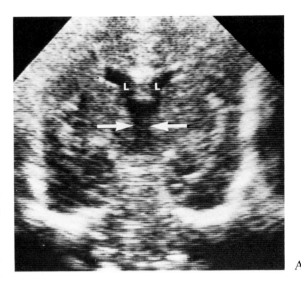

A

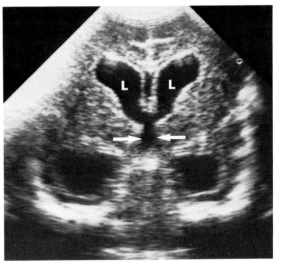

B

FIGURE 4-20. Coronal sections from neonates with PVL and atrophy (**A**) and PHH (**B**). PVL and atrophy result in equal enlargement of lateral ventricles and third ventricle. PHH causes relatively greater expansion of lateral ventricles (*L*) when compared to third ventricle (*arrows*).

Widening of the cerebral sulci and enlargement of the subarachnoid space are the external signs of cerebral wasting. Internally, this same wasting affects the ventricular system, another expandable CSF space. As the brain shrinks, the ventricles enlarge, resulting in ex vacuuo hydrocephalus. In our experience, close observation reveals a unique ventricular configuration in these children. The frontal horns are often somewhat more enlarged than the posterior

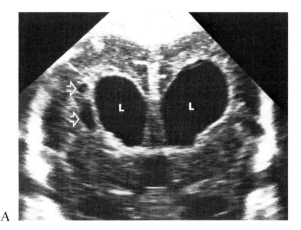

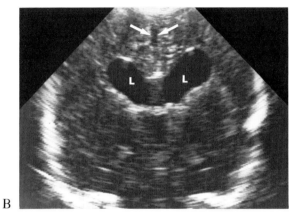

FIGURE 4-21. Coronal scans in same patient before (**A**) and after (**B**) ventricular decompression by shunt. Lateral ventricles (*L*) have decreased in size, and cystic PVL lateral to right ventricle (*open arrows*) is no longer visible in **B**. Note widening of interhemispheric fissure in **B** (*arrows*), which was not present before relief of increased intracranial pressure. (From Grant EG, Schellinger D, 1985.[16])

portions of the lateral ventricles, and the third ventricle is enlarged to a similar mild degree as the lateral ventricles. These findings are never present in children with pure posthemorrhagic hydrocephalus (PHH). In PHH, the occipital horns and trigones are always the most severely affected parts of the ventricular system. Additionally, in PHH, the lateral ventricles are always markedly enlarged before the third ventricle is even affected. This is not the case in atrophy; the third and lateral ventricles are enlarged to a similar degree, as might be expected from a global process (Fig. 4-20 A and B).

The sonographic findings indicative of atrophy may be obliterated by PHH. The subtle ventricular changes are obviously obscured, and the cerebral sulci may be compressed from increased intracranial pressure. Similar to the findings in a child with cystic PVL who has reverted to a normal sonogram but continues to have underlying scarring, the sonographic findings of atrophy are only masked by hydrocephalus. The pathology remains; two of three patients developed obvious widening of the interhemispheric fissure after decompression of the hydrocephalus by shunting (Fig. 4-21 A and B).

The significance of atrophy in infants already burdened with PVL remains to be investigated. Certainly, many of the abnormalities described in the pathology literature point to a diffuse cerebral insult in addition to localized periventricular infarction. We must, however, continue to depend on the older literature for such information, since little data is yet available from present ICN populations.

References

1. Little WJ. Course of lectures on the deformities of the human frame: Lecture VIII. Lancet I:318–322, 1843.
2. Virchow R. Zur pathologischen anatomie des gehirns: 1. Congenitale encephalitis und myelitis. Virchow Arch Pathol Anat 38:129–142, 1867.
3. Parrot JM. Etude sur le ramollissement de l'encephale chez le nouveau-ne'. Arch Physiol Norm Pathol (Paris) 5:59–73, 1873.
4. Parrot JM. Etude sur le ramollissement de l'encephale chez le nouveau-ne'. Arch Physiol Norm Pathol (Paris) 5:176–195, 1873.
5. Parrot JM. Etude sur le ramollissement de l'encephale chez le nouveau-ne.' Arch Physiol Norm Pathol (Paris) 5:283–303, 1873.
6. Banker BQ, Larroche JC. Periventricular leukomalacia of infancy. Arch Neurol 7:386–409, 1962.
7. DiChiro G, Arimitsu T, Pellock JM, Landes RD. Periventricular leukomalacia related to neonatal anoxia: recognition by computed tomography. J Comput Assist Tomogr 2:352–355, 1978.
8. Hill A, Melson GL, Clark HB, Volpe JJ. Hemorrhagic periventricular leukomalacia: diagnosis by real-time ultrasound and correlation with autopsy findings. Pediatrics 69:282–284, 1982.
9. Grant EG, Schellinger D, Richardson JD, Coffey ML, Smirniotopoulos JG. Echogenic periventricular halo: normal sonographic findings or neonatal cerebral hemorrhage. AJNR 4:43–46, 1983.

10. Levene MI, Wigglesworth JS, Dubowitz V. Hemorrhagic periventricular leukomalacia in the neonate: a real-time ultrasound study. Pediatrics 71:794–797, 1983.

11. DeReuck J, Chattha AS, Richardson EP. Pathogenesis and evolution of periventricular leukomalacia in infancy. Arch Neurol 27:229–236, 1972.

12. Armstrong D, Norman MG. Periventricular leukomalacia in neonates: complications and sequelae. Arch Dis Child 49:367–375, 1974.

13. Shuman RM, Selednik LJ, Periventricular leukomalacia: a one-year autopsy study. Arch Neurol 37:231–235, 1980.

14. Schellinger D, Grant EG, Richardson JD. Cystic periventricular leukomalacia: sonographic and CT findings. AJNR 5:439–445, 1984.

15. Grant EG, Schellinger D. Periventricular leukomalacia in combination with intraventricular hemorrhage: sonographic features and sequelae. AJNR (in press).

16. Grant EG, Schellinger D. Sonography of neonatal periventricular leukomalacia: recent experience with a 7.5-MHz scanner. AJNR 6:781–785, 1985. Williams & Wilkins.

17. Babcock DS, Ball W. Postaphyxial encephalopathy in full-term infants: ultrasound diagnosis. Radiology 148:417–423, 1983.

5
Incidence and Outcome: Germinal Matrix-Related Hemorrhage

Yolande F. Smith

Incidence and Outcome of Intraventricular Hemorrhage in the Premature Infant

"We dissected the head of the fourth child which died within the first month . . . in the cavity below the cerebellum, immediately above the trunk of the medulla oblongata, we found a considerable quantity of gumous blood."—Thomas Willis, 1667.[1] This, the first account of neonatal intracranial hemorrhage in the seventeenth century, left its author with as many questions as we have today, 300 years later.

It was Gruenwald[2] in 1951, reporting in the Journal of Obstetrics and Gynecology, who first made the association between subependymal hemorrhage and prematurity. Over the next 20 years, with the early advances in neonatal care accounting for better survival in the sick premature, germinal matrix-related hemorrhage (GMRH) became one of the major causes of death in low-birthweight infants. Investigators naturally turned to autopsy data in an effort to elucidate its incidence, pathology, and pathogenesis. Incidence figures ranged from 20% to 70%[3-7] among premature infants subject to autopsy; in addition, Harcke et al.,[7] in 1972, recognized the inverse relationship between gestational age (GA) and GMRH, and also the increasing incidence in the first 72 hr of life (a threefold increase from 23% in infants dying within the first 24 hr to 73% in those who died between 24 and 72 hr). In 1977, the first epidemiologic survey of perinatal intracranial hemorrhage was reported by Schoenberg et al.[8] as a record review of births in the Rochester population for 1965–1974; he estimated the incidence as 1 per 1,000 live births, but failed to give the general incidence of prematurity in the population.

In 1978, Papile et al.[9] prospectively utilized computed tomography (CT) in 46 infants weighing less than 1500 g at birth and reported a 43% occurrence of GMRH. Their most startling finding, however, was that 78% of their infants with GMRH had no symptomatology referable to the GMRH—a diagnosis that previously was sought only in infants with severe neurologic compromise.

The introduction of portable cranial ultrasonography in the past 5 years has facilitated the diagnosis of GMRH[10-12] and helped to intensify interest in this enigmatic disease. Most tertiary care neonatal units now routinely employ this method as a screening tool. Consequently, there are numerous reports on the incidence of GMRH, ranging from 30% to 90% in the premature population with a median range of 40–50%. Many factors[13-19] have been implicated for the variation in incidence: socioeconomic conditions, inborn versus transport, prenatal drug administration (e.g., steroids and betamimetics); however, none of these have been well substantiated by other investigators.

In our own Intensive Care Nursery population at Georgetown University Hospital, of 163 infants admitted from January 1980 through December 1981 that weighed 1750 g or less at birth at a gestational age of 34 weeks or less, the incidence was 52% (85 of 163). Two-thirds of our infants were inborn; one-third were transported from smaller referring institutions. Inci-

TABLE 5-1. Incidence of GMRH: 1980–1981

Birthweight (g)	Number of infants admitted	Number of infants with sonogram	Normal	GMRH	GMRH (%)
501–750	20	16	2	14	70
751–1250	68	63	16	47	70
1251–1750	75	58	34	24	32
Total:	163	137	52	85	52

dence varied inversely with gestational age (and birthweight): Infants under 30 weeks gestation (and <1251 g) had double the incidence of those delivered between 31 and 34 weeks.

Twenty-six infants did not have sonograms: Nine infants weighed 1250 g or less at birth and died within 24 hr; of these, six infants had autopsy evidence of GMRH. One infant weighed 1450 g and died at 2 days of age; no evidence of hemorrhage was found on autopsy. The other 16 infants weighed 1501–1750 g, were all healthy, and were transferred to the Intermediate Care Nursery after a short observation period (<24 hr), thus eluding the routine cranial sonographic screening done in the Intensive Care Nursery.

Bejar et al[14] reported a 41% incidence of minor (Grades I and II) hemorrhages and a 49% occurrence of major (Grades III and IV) hemorrhages in a population comparable to ours. Papile et al.[17] and Pape et al.,[10] on the other hand, in separate studies found a greater incidence of minor bleeds (Grades I and II) in their populations (60% minor versus 40% major).

The severity of hemorrhages in our population was distributed as in Table 5-2.

In 1981[20] we reported a 43% progression of GMRH between the initial sonogram done within the first 2 days of life and a follow-up study done between days 3 and 7. Twenty-seven of 51 (53%) infants studied had stable

sonographic findings, while 22 (43%) progressed to a higher grade hemorrhage. This is in keeping with the data of Tsiantos et al.,[21] Harcke et al.,[7] and other authors, who estimated that the commonest time of the actual hemorrhage was about 2–3 days of age as a sequel to the perinatal insult.

Survival

Survival statistics for the study period 1980–1981 ranged from 30% in infants weighing 750 g or less to 92% in infants weighing 1251–1750 g at birth.

The occurrence of intraventricular hemorrhage (IVH) significantly decreased survival in the total study group, from 94% in infants without IVH to 65% in infants with IVH. In contrast to other reports,[17,22] there was no difference in survival between infants with minor or major hemorrhages (see Table 5-3).

Complications

Hydrocephalus has long been recognized as a sequel of neonatal intraventricular hemorrhage.[9,16,22–24] Thirty (54%) of the surviving infants with IVH had sonographic evidence of ventricular dilatation by 3 weeks of age. Only one infant with Grade I developed ventricular distension, but 50% of infants with Grades II and III hemorrhages [8 (40%) of 20 with Grade II and 13 (62%) of 21 with Grade III] had evi-

TABLE 5-2. Severity of hemorrhage in relation to birth weight

Birthweight (g)	I	II	III	IV
501–750	4	6	3	1
751–1250	4	14	18	11
1251–1750	1	7	8	8
Total infants	9	27	29	20
Total GMRH (%)	10	32	34	24

(Highest grade of hemorrhage)

TABLE 5-3. IVH grading and survival

Sonogram	Normal	I	II	III	IV
Number of infants	52	9	27	29	20
Survivors	49	5	20	21	10
Survival (%)	94	55	74	72	50

(Grade)

TABLE 5-4. Follow-up group

	Grade IVH				
	Normal	I	II	III	IV
Survivors	49	5	20	21	10
Follow-up to 18 months	23 (47%)	5 (100%)	12 (60%)	17 (81%)	7 (70%)
Mean gestational age (wks)	29.95	29.0	28.5	28.9	29.1[a]
Mean birthweight (g)	1237	1121	1022	1168	1184

[a] Not statistically significant.

dence of mild to moderate dilatation. Eight (80%) of 10 infants with Grade IV GMRH had moderate to severe hydrocephalus. In 1980, all infants having evidence of ventricular distension were treated with alternate-day spinal taps[24, 26] and re-evaluated with follow-up sonograms. In view of the fact that all but two infants resolved their ventriculomegaly in 10–14 days, in 1981 we discontinued the use of serial spinal taps (LP). There were five exceptions; these were infants who had progressive ventricular dilatation on two or more serial weekly cranial sonograms. Shankaran et al.[27] have since reported no significant difference in the number of infants requiring shunt insertion in LP- and non-LP-treated groups.

Three infants (one with Grade III and two with Grade IV) had placement of ventricular reservoirs for noncommunicating hydrocephalus; these were tapped three times weekly, but were all subsequently converted to ventriculoperitoneal shunts. Porencephalic cysts[28, 29] developed in all of the surviving infants with Grade IV hemorrhage. In a number of infants with small porencephalic cysts and decompressed ventricles, the cysts were not visible on late follow-up sonograms. Large defects, however, persisted on follow-up sonograms and/or CT scans for as long as these children were followed.

Developmental Outcome

After discharge, all infants are followed in the Developmental Evaluation Clinic and seen by a multidisciplinary team of developmental pediatricians, child psychologists, physical and occupational therapists, audiologists, and other support personnel. Infants are seen at 3, 6, 9, 12, 18, and 24 months chronological age, and at each visit are evaluated by standard neurologic

criteria and by Bayley Scales of Motor (PDI) and Mental (MDI) Development. Speech and hearing tests are also administered at 1 year of age. Bayley scores are corrected for gestational age; scores less than 84 are considered abnormal, and scores of 84 or more are considered normal.

Sixty-four (64%) of the 105 survivors studied by cranial ultrasonography were seen regularly for the first 2 years (Table 5-4).

Follow-up was more diligent in hemorrhage survivors (73%) than in nonhemorrhage survivors, probably reflecting both parenteral anxiety about the hemorrhage and also the intensity to which the staff pursued infants with documented hemorrhage. Mean age at follow-up was 22 months (range, 17–30 months).

Birthweight and gestational age were not significantly different among the five groups (mean GA, 29.2 weeks; mean birthweight, 1164 g). The data are summarized in Table 5-5.

Infants without Evidence of GMRH

Of the 23 infants evaluated, only 1 had severe neurodevelopmental delay. (This infant's

TABLE 5-5. Outcome of premature infants with or without GMRH

	Grade of GMRH				
	None	I	II	III	IV
Normal[a]	83	40	67	47	43
Mild neurodevelopmental impairment[b]	13	40	8	35	14
Severe neurodevelopmental impairment[c]	4	20	25	18	43
Number of infants	23	5	12	17	7

[a] Normal neurologic evaluation, PDI and MDI greater than 84. Data are percentages.
[b] One parameter abnormal, two parameters normal (Neuro, PDI, MDI). Data are percentages.
[c] Two or three abnormal parameters. Data are percentages.

course was complicated by many factors known to correlate with poor outcome, i.e., low maternal age, lack of prenatal care, precipitious delivery, severe perinatal asphyxia, and neonatal seizures.) The three infants with mild impairment were only moderately delayed on either the MDI or PDI, and had normal neurologic evaluations. For the entire group, the mean motor score (PDI) was 97.1 (range, 50–119) and the mean mental score was 107.2 (range, 60–150) at 24 months, with 22 of 23 infants neurologically normal.

Infants with Grade I GMRH

Two of five infants in this group were normal on follow-up; three infants had mild hyperreflexia, but in only one of these infants did this cause a functional motor delay as evidenced by a low PDI (69). All infants had normal mental evaluations, with a mean score of 107.3 (range, 96–114) and a mean PDI of 100.0 (range, 69–124).

Infants with Grade II GMRH

Significant neurodevelopmental delay was present in 3 of the 12 infants followed. One infant was multiply handicapped (including severe visual impairment), and the other two had normal mental evaluations with some evidence of motor deficits. One infant continued to have mild generalized hypertonia, although developmental assessments were normal. Eight infants are functioning within normal limits. Mean PDI was 98.5 (73–116), and mean MDI 102.1 (62–140), at 2 years of age.

Infants with Grade III GMRH

Almost half of these infants were normal at 2-year follow-up (8 of 17). Four infants had residual neurologic abnormalities (three with mild hypertonia and one with extrapyramidal palsy) but they all functioned within normal limits developmentally. Two infants had low Bayley motor scores at 14 and 17 months, with normal mental and neurologic evaluations. Unfortunately, they have both been lost to follow-up, but all the other infants whom we have seen with this pattern (abnormal motor, normal mental and neuro) at 12 months (9–17) have normal

motor scores by 2 years of age. Three infants (including one with a V-P shunt) had multiple handicaps and required special school programs in their third year of life. Mean PDI was 97.4 (range, <50–131), and MDI was 104.2 (range, 56–150).

Infants with Intraparenchymal (Grade IV) Hemorrhage

Of seven infants followed, one infant is severely delayed, two have significant motor handicaps with normal mental evaluations, and three infants were functioning normally at 2 years of age. One infant demonstrated persistent hypotonia at 30 months of age, but had normal Bayley scores.

Infants with Shunts

Three infants, one infant with Grade III hemorrhage and two infants with Grade IV, had V-P shunts. Two of those infants (one with Grade III and one with Grade IV) are multiple handicapped; one infant has spastic quadriplegia, but is mentally normal; the other infant is functioning normally at 25 months of age with motor and mental scores of 114 and 116 and normal neurologic evaluation. This infant's only problems are visual (i.e., strabismus and myopia requiring eyeglasses).

Earlier studies suggested that the presence of GMRH was a poor prognostic indicator of neurodevelopmental outcome. More recently, Papile et al.,[17] Koons et al.,[30] Ment et al.,[31] and other authors have more encouraging reports, and relate handicaps to the severity of GMRH and its complications. In our population, consistent with other investigators, neurodevelopmental delay is proportional to the magnitude of the hemorrhage (and probably a reflection of the hypoxic/ischemic insult); however, we are very encouraged that infants with major hemorrhages (Grades III and IV) still have a 45% chance of normal outcome. Even more heartening is the low incidence of mental impairment, even when motor handicaps prevail. In our sample, too, a normal Bayley mental evaluation (even with abnormal motor) at 12 months of age was predictive of a normal overall outcome at 2 years of age. Further follow-up is necessary to look for preschool and early schoolage problems to which these patients are susceptible, but certainly in 1985 we can be more optimistic in counseling parents of premature infants with GMRH.

References

1. Willis T. Pathologiae Cerebri et Nervosi Generis Specimen, In quo Agitur de Morbis Convulsivis, et de Scorbuto. Oxomi, execudebat Guil Hall, impensis Ja Allestry, p 49, 1167.
2. Greenwald P. Subependymal cerebral hemorrhage in premature infants and its relation to various injurious influences at birth. Am J Obstet Gynecol 61:1285, 1951.
3. Towbin A. Cerebral intraventricular hemorrhage and subependymal matrix infarction in the fetus and premature newborn. Am J Pathol 52:121, 1968.
4. Valdes-Dapena MA, Arey JB. The causes of neonatal mortality: an analysis of 501 autopsies on newborn infants. J Pediatr 77:366, 1970.
5. Frederick J, Butler MR. Certain causes of neonatal death. II. Intraventricular hemorrhage. Biol Neonate 15:257, 1970.
6. Wigglesworth JS, Dame PA, Keith IH, Stade SA. Intraventricular hemorrhage in the preterm infant without hyaline membrane disease. Arch Dis Child 52:447, 1977.
7. Harcke HT, Naeye RL, Storch A, Blanc WA. Perinatal cerebral intraventricular hemorrhage. J Pediatr 80:37, 1972.
8. Schoenberg BS, Mellinger JF, Schoenberg DG. Perinatal intracranial hemorrhage. Arch Neurol 34:570, 1977.
9. Papile L, Burnstein J, Burnstein R, Koffler H. Incidence and evolution of supependymal and intraventricular hemorrhage: A study of infants with birth weights less than 1500 gm. J Pediatr 92:529, 1978.
10. Pape RE, Lusich G, Houang MTW, Blackwell RJ, Sherwood A, Thorburn RJ, Reynolds EDR. Ultrasound detection of brain damage in preterm infants. Lancet I:1261, 1979.
11. Johnson ML, Rumack CM. Ultrasonic evaluation of the neonatal brain. Radiol Clin North Am 18:117, 1980.
12. Grant EG, Schellinger D, Borts FT, McCullough DC, Friedman GR, Siva Subramanian KN, Smith YF. Real-time ultrasonography of the neonatal head. Am J Neuroradiol 1(6):487, 1980.
13. Clark CE, Clymann RI, Roth RS, Sniderman SH, Lane B, Ballard RA. Risk factor analysis of intraventricular hemorrhage in low birth weight infants. J Pediatr 99:625, 1981.
14. Bejar P, Curbelo B, Coen RW, Leopold G,

15. James H, Gluck L. Diagnosis and follow-up of intraventricular and intracerebral hemorrhages by ultrasound studies of infant's brain through the fontanelles and sutures. Pediatrics 66:661, 1980.
15. Levene MI, Wigglesworth JS, Dubowitz V. Cerebral structure and intraventricular hemorrhage in the neonate: a real-time ultrasound study. Arch Dis Child 56:416, 1981.
16. Ahmann PA, Lazzara A, Dykes F, Brann AW, Schwartz J. Intraventricular hemorrhage in the high-risk preterm infant: incidence and outcome. Ann Neurol 7:118, 1980.
17. Papile L, Munsick-Bruno A, Schaefer A. Relationship of cerebral intraventricular hemorrhage and early childhood neurologic handicaps. J Pediatr 103:273, 1983.
18. Horbar JD, Pasnich M, McAuliffe TL, Lucey JF. Obstetrical factors and the risk of periventricular–intraventricular hemorrhage in infants weighing less than 1200 gms at birth. The Second Special Ross Laboratory Conference on Perinatal Intracranial Hemorrhage, Syllabus, 339, 1982.
19. Lazzara A, Kanto WP, Dykes FD, Ahmann PA, West K. Continuing education in the community hospital and reduction in the incidence of intracerebral hemorrhage in the transported preterm infant. J Pediatr 101:757, 1982.
20. Smith YF, Siva Subramanian KN, Davitt MK, Grant EG, McCullough D. Progression of intraventricular hemorrhage in premature infants. Pediatr Res 16:308A,
21. Tsiantos A, Victorin L, Relies JP, Nyer N, Sindell H, Brill AB, Stahlman M. Intracranial hemorrhage in the prematurely born infant. J Pediatr 85:854, 1974.
22. Volpe JJ. Intracranial hemorrhage in the newborn: current understanding and dilemmas. Neurology 29:632, 1979.
23. Larroche JC. Post-hemorrhagic hydrocephalus in infancy: anatomical study. Biol Neonate 20:287, 1972.
24. Deonna T, Payot M, Probst A, Prodham LS. Neonatal intracranial hemorrhage in premature infants. Pediatrics 56:1056, 1975.
25. Goldstein GW, Chapling ER, Maitland J, Normand D. Transient hydrocephalus in premature infants: Treatment by lumbar puncture. Lancet I:512, 1976.
26. Papile L, Burnstein J, Burnstein R, Koffler H, Koops BL, Johnson JD. Post-hemorrhagic hydrocephalus in low birthweight infants: Treatment by serial lumbar punctures. J Pediatr 97:272, 1980.
27. Shankaran S, Bedard MP, Slovis TL, The changing incidence of periventricular–intraventricular hemorrhage. The Second Special Ross Laborato-

ries Conference on Perinatal Intracranial Hemorrhage, Syllabus, 1012, 1982.

28. Smith YF, Siva Subramanian KN, Davitt MK,
McCullough D, Grant E, Borts F. Use of ultrasound in the diagnosis of intracerebral hemorrhage and porencephalic cyst in neonates. Presented at Third World Congress and 10th Annual
SCCM Meeting on Critical Care Medicine, May
1981.

29. Grant EG, Schellinger D, Borts F, McCullough
D, Siva Subramanian KN, Smith YF, Davitt
MK. Evolution of porencephalic cysts from in-
traparenchymal hemorrhage in neonates. Am J
Neuroadiol. 3:47, 1982.

30. Koons A, Sum S, Kamtorn V, Hagorsky M,
Koenigsberger R. Neurodevelopmental outcome
related to intraventricular hemorrhage and perinatal events. The Second Special Ross Laboratories Conference on Perinatal Intracranial Hemorrhage, Syllabus, page 1065, 1982.

31. Ment R, Scott DT, Ehrenkranz RA, Warshaw
JB. Follow-up of very low birthweight (VLBW)
infants: Late developmental sequelae in GMH/
IVH survivors. The Second Special Ross Labo-
ratories Conference on Perinatal Intracranial
Hemorrhage, Syllabus, page 1117, 1982.

6
Incidence and Outcome: Periventricular Leukomalacia

Yolande F. Smith

Periventricular Leukomalacia in the Neonate

Incidence

The introduction of portable cranial sonography[1-3] into intensive care neonatal units during the past 5 years has not only facilitated the diagnosis of intraventricular hemorrhage (IVH), but has also helped to intensify interest in neonatal intracranial disease as a whole.

Periventricular leukomalacia (PVL) has been described by many authors from neonatal postmortem studies. Its frequency is assessed at 7–18%,[4-7] with a predilection for infants with a birthweight of 900–2200 g who have survived more than 6 days. However, the "in vivo" diagnosis of PVL by cranial sonography[8-10] has only recently been described, so that prospective studies on its incidence in infants at risk are limited. Levine et al., in their British study,[8] reported an incidence of 7.5% in infants with birthweights of 1,500 g or less, consistent with the 6.4% incidence in infants weighing 1750 g or less at birth admitted to our Intensive Care Nursery at Georgetown University Hospital.

The birthweights of the affected infants in our population ranged from 680 to 1730 g, with a mean weight of 1247 g ($\pm$98 SD). Gestational age varied from 26 to 33 weeks, and all infants had birthweights appropriate for gestational age (mean, 29.12 $\pm$ 2.09 SD) (see Table 6-1).

PVL was diagnosed most commonly in the first week of life (64%, 16 of 25 infants), including 9 infants (36%) in whom the diagnosis was apparent as early as the first sonogram within the first 72 hr. However, PVL emerged as late as 7 weeks in two infants with previously normal studies up to 2 weeks of age.

There were bilateral lesions in 21 infants (84%), right-sided in 3, and left-sided in 1 infant. The lesions were spread among most of the ventricular margin in the majority (92%) of infants, but was localized to the frontal area in two infants (one bilateral, one unilateral).

Twenty infants had sonographic evidence of intraventricular blood in addition to PVL, but the origin of the hemorrhage could not be differentiated as being either from the periventricular infarct or the accompanying germinal matrix bleed.

The presence of PVL did not alter survival in our population: Infants with PVL had a survival rate of 80% (20 of 25), not significantly different from the infants without PVL in the study group (83.3%) (see Table 6-1).

Outcome

Motor Development

All 16 infants with PVL who survived 12 months or more have been evaluated using standard developmental criteria.[11, 12] Fourteen have severe motor deficits at 12–25 months (mean, 15 months) of the spastic variety. One infant with PVL localized to the right frontal area has a normal corrected PDI of 92 at 12 months, but on neurologic evaluation, she demonstrated hypertonia of both lower limbs (see Table 6-2).

The 6-month motor evaluation was very misleading in this group of infants. Nine of the 16

TABLE 6-1. Characteristics of study group (PVL vs. no PVL)

	Birthweight (g) (mean ± SD)	Gestational age (weeks) (mean ± SD)	IVH (%)	Survival (%)
Infants with PVL (n = 25)	1247 ± 98	29.12 ± 2.07	80	80
Infants without PVL (n = 364)	1199 ± 110	28.8 ± 1.98	52	83.3

infants evaluated had motor Bayley scores within the normal range at 6 months; however, only 1 of these remained normal on 12-month follow-up. The other eight infants showed either arrest or deterioration of motor development between 6 and 12 months of age. None of the four infants with delayed motor function at 6–9 months improved toward the end of the first year.

Mental Development

Four of the 16 infants surviving 12 months or more have normal mental function by Bayley evaluation. Consistent with the pattern seen with motor evaluation, the 6-month evaluation was not a good predictor of later function; only 4 of 10 infants with a normal mental score at 6 months tested within the normal range at 1 year (see Table 6-2).

The neurological evaluation was abnormal in all our infants. Spastic diplegia or quadriplegia were the most common findings. These diagno-

TABLE 6-2. Neurodevelopmental outcome of 16 infants with PVL[a]

	Number of infants	Percent of total
Neurologic sequelae:		
Spastic quadriplegia	10	62.5
Spastic diplegia	4	25.0
Lower limb hypertonia	1	6.25
Mild left hemiplegia	1	6.25
Truncal hypotonia	14	87.5
Poor head control	14	87.5
Cortical blindness	6	37.5
Bayley evaluation:		
Abnormal MDI (<84, corrected for GA)[b]	12	75.0
Abnormal PDI (<84, corrected for GA)[b]	14	87.5

[a] Infants older than 12 months (range, 12–25).
[b] GA, Gestational age.

ses were based on increased tone, especially in the adductor motor groups: hyperactive deep-tendon reflexes; the presence of ankle clonus; fisting of hands; scissoring of legs; and impaired ability to support weight. In addition, poor truncal tone and poor head control were present in all but one infant over one year of age. The two infants with mild neurological symptoms exhibited hypertonia of both lower extremities (left more so than right) with increased deep-tendon reflexes, but no scissoring or ankle clonus. Examination of the upper extremities was within normal limits. On cranial ultrasonography, these infants' lesions were localized to the right frontal area.

Outcome of Infants Less Than 12 Months

Four additional PVL survivors are now less than 1 year of age. In accordance with the pattern of their older counterparts, they all have abnormal neurological findings of the spastic variety, with resulting low Bayley motor scores (except one). Mental performance is so far within normal limits in 3 of the 4 infants. It is interesting to note that the single infant with normal Bayley mental and motor evaluations also shows focal frontal PVL.

The clinical sequelae of PVL as typified by our population were very accurately described by W.J. Little[13] in 1843: " . . . mental retardation and spasticity of all the limbs . . . the spasticity was not always symmetrical, and the legs were more severely afflicted than the arms . . . "

Although larger and longer-term studies are necessary to fully define the clinical antecedents and sequelae of PVL, we postulate from our limited 2-year follow-up that the presence of this entity is an extremely poor prognostic sign in the sick preterm infant. Every effort should be made in the perinatal period to prevent the cerebral hypoperfusion that appears to herald this disease.

References

1. Grant EG, Garrett WJ, Radavanovich G. Ultrasonic atlas of normal brain of infant. Med Biol 1:259–266, 1974.
2. Grant EG, Borts FT, Schellinger D, McCullough DC, Siva Subramanian KN, Smith Y. Real-time ultrasonography of neonatal intraventricular hemorrhage and comparison with computed tomography. Radiology 139:687–691. 1981.
3. Haber K, Wachter RD, Christenson PC, Vaucher Y, Sahn DJ, Smith JR. Ultrasonic evaluation of intracranial pathology in infants: a new technique. Radiology 134:173–178, 1980.
4. Armstrong D, Norman MG. Periventricular leukomalacia in neonates: complications and sequelae. Arch Dis Child 49:367–375, 1974.
5. Banker BQ, Larroche JC. Periventricular leukomalacia of infancy: a form of neonatal anoxic encephalopathy. Arch Neurol 7:386–410, 1962.
6. Shuman RM, Selednik LJ. Periventricular leukomalacia: a one-year autopsy study. Arch Neurol 37:231–235, 1980.
7. De Rueck J, Chattha AS, Richardson EP Jr. Pathogenesis and evolution of periventricular leukomalacia. Arch Neurol 27:229–236, 1972.
8. Levine MI, Wigglesworth JS, Dubowitz V. Hemorrhagic periventricular leukomalacia in the neonate: a real-time ultrasound study. Pediatrics 71:794–797, 1983.
9. Hill A, Martin DJ, Daneman A, Fitz CR. Focal ischemic cerebral injury in the newborn: diagnosis by ultrasound and correlation with computed tomographic scan. Pediatrics 71:790–793, 1983.
10. Grant EG, Schellinger D, Richardson JD, Coffey ML, Smirniotopolous JG. Echogenic periventricular halo: normal sonographic finding of neonatal cerebral hemorrhage. AJNR 4:43–46, 1983.
11. Bayley N. Manual for the Bayley Scales of Infant Development. New York, Psychological Corporation, 1969.
12. Amiel-Tison C. A method for neurological evaluation within the first year of life. In: Current Problems in Pediatrics, Vol. III, No. 1. Gluck L, ed. Chicago, Yearbook Medical Publishers, 1976.
13. Little WJ. Course of lectures on the deformities of the human frame: Lecture VIII. Lancet I:318–322, 1843.

7
Comparison of Two Modalities: Ultrasound versus Computed Tomography

Dieter Schellinger

Introduction

If one compares the diagnostic spectrum and efficacy of two competing imaging methods, a multitude of objectives need to be assessed; these include degree of invasiveness, ease of performance, cost, and associated noxious effects as well as accuracy, sensitivity, and specificity. While several of these items can be addressed squarely and unequivocally, others are more difficult to discuss. There is copious literature on the accuracy of computed tomography (CT), including large autopsy series.[2, 5, 38, 39] There are also sufficient literature data concerning clinical comparison of sonography and CT, particularly on intracerebral hemorrhage and ventricular dilatation. However, fewer data are available on ultrasonic clinicopathologic correlations, and at this writing there are no major series of postmortem ultrasound–CT comparisons. Nevertheless, there are sufficient clinical observations in the literature to permit a general comparison of the two modalities. In the course of this discussion, we will also refer to our own clinical experiences.

To judge the global diagnostic impact of either modality, it is important to consider which of the various disease categories in the neonatal age group most significantly impact immediate survival and long-term neurodevelopmental outcome. We believe this merits a detailed discussion before we present a direct comparison.

Neonatal Cerebral Pathologies and Their Early and Long-Term Effects on Neurodevelopmental Outcome

Neonatal Death

Between 31% and 41%[1, 2, 3] of very preterm infants or neonates with perinatal asphyxia will not survive. Necropsy studies on diseased neonates show intracerebral hemorrhage as the leading abnormality,[5, 18] with an incidence of 43–86%.[3, 4, 6] Ischemic changes in the form of periventricular leukomalacia or infarcts are reported to occur in 7–57% of diseased infants[2, 69–72] and among 87% of expired neonates with intraventricular hemorrhage.[7] There is also a broad concensus among authors[1, 2, 8] about the impact of intracranial hemorrhage on mortality. Stewart[1] places the mortality of low-grade intracranial hemorrhage (Grade I–II) at 15–46% and that of high-grade intracranial hemorrhage (Grade III–IV) at 55–69%.

Surviving Neonates

In the group of neonatal survivors, intracranial hemorrhage again leads the statistics with an incidence of 40–60%.[3, 9] Data on frequency of ischemic brain damage are based on small case materials. The reported range of 4.5–7%[4, 10] is probably too low, as is discussed later.[73]

There is a direct relationship between the severity of intracranial hemorrhage and the incidence of ventriculomegaly.[11] A similar correlation exists relative to the development of late neurodevelopmental handicaps.[12-17] In two series,[1,3] higher grade intracranial hemorrhage signaled adverse neurodevelopmental outcome in 50-54%. The presence of ventriculomegaly is an even more penetrant factor, as it denotes handicap in 71%. Neurologic sequelae are higher in advanced ventriculomegaly (75%), and less common in mild ventricular dilatation (38%). In one series, ventricular enlargement, when associated with cerebral atrophy, had an adverse outcome in all patients studied.[1]

All available data emphasize the impact of intracranial hemorrhage on immediate survival and late neurodevelopmental outcome. They also point out the importance of ventricular enlargement, which, either alone or with intracranial hemorrhage, is the single most important predictor for evolving neurodevelopmental handicap.[1]

A major cause of ventriculomegaly is intracerebral hemorrhage, but a sizeable group of patients develop ventriculomegaly ex vacuo without preceding intracranial hemorrhage. Documentable cortical atrophy may account for some, whereas loss of white matter mass, either secondary to periventricular leukomalacia or to infarcts, may offer the most plausible explanation for others.

An interesting group of handicapped survivors have either no documentable cerebral abnormalities (8%) or only Grade I intracranial hemorrhage (8-46%).[1,3] Cerebral ischemia may be a major etiologic factor in these patients.

It appears safe to state that the major cerebral pathologies, early or late, are those of intracranial hemorrhage and/or cerebral ischemia. Consequently, accurate assessment of brain parenchyma and cerebrospinal fluid (CSF) spaces with recognition of hemorrhagic as well as ischemic cerebral pathologies is paramount in neonatal brain imaging.

Ventricles

The diagnosis of ventricular enlargement is similar in importance to intracranial hemorrhage, since both have important prognostic implica-tions. The two pathologies frequently interdigitate: Virtually all forms of intracranial hemorrhage may ultimately lead to ventriculomegaly. Long-range sequelae of ventriculomegaly were discussed earlier.

Ventricular enlargement may follow the pathodynamics of ex vacuo or obstructive hydrocephalus. Loss of brain mass may lead to ventricular expansion. Subarachnoid hemorrhage can cause arachnoiditis with blockage of CSF pathways and absorptive surfaces. Obstruction at the ventricular level, secondary to blood clots or ependymitis, is a frequent cause of ventricular expansion.

Both CT and sonography have been found accurate in evaluating hydrocephalus.[18-22] This is also supported by an autopsy series.[18] As CT usually produces a more complete cross-sectional image, it is easier to show the complexity of ventricular abnormalities, especially in patients with congenital cerebral abnormalities (Fig. 7-1). Normal-sized fourth ventricles are not routinely delineated on axial sonographic cuts. Sagittal views may be needed for identification. Occasionally, ventricular septa can be encountered. These represent postinflammatory changes, and may follow ventriculitis or ependymitis secondary to ventricular hemorrhage. These are easily missed with CT, and can be better appreciated with sonography (Fig. 7-2).

Ultrasound has the advantage of presenting the ventricles in at least two planes. The frontal and temporal horns can be observed in a coronal, semiaxial, and angled sagittal view. Ventricular bodies and trigonal areas are viewed in semiaxial and angled sagittal planes. Because of the greater complexity of the test, CT scanning in neonates is usually performed in the axial plane only. Occasionally, parts of the ventricular system may not be included on routine CT cuts. Therefore, ultrasound provides a more complex picture of the ventricular system. The trigonal areas of the lateral ventricles are the most sensitive anatomic regions for early ventricular expansion. Ventricular measurements with ultrasound and CT, therefore, must take this into account.

The routinely performed multidirectional scanning with ultrasound allows for a more complete depiction of the ventricular perimeter, including the ventricular lining. This shows

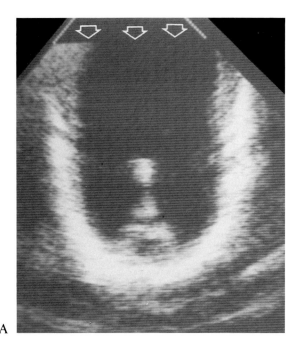

A

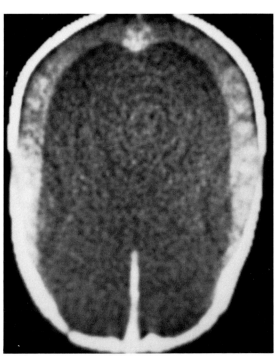

B

FIGURE 7-1. Ventricular size is accurately gauged by CT and ultrasound. However, CT more precisely depicts borders of ventricles and shows entire axial plane. Ultrasound, because of the near-field artifacts, may miss the anterior portion. **A**, Sonogram showing expanded lateral ventricles in patient with congenital hydrocephalus. Frontal portion cut off (*arrows*) because of necessity of scanning through anterior fontanelle. **B**, CT of same patient. Expanded lateral ventricles more completely delineated and margins more precisely defined. Frontal portion fully included on scan.

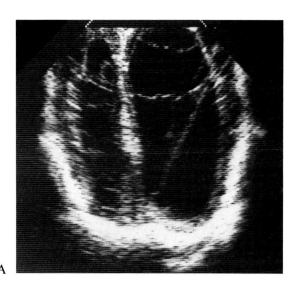

A

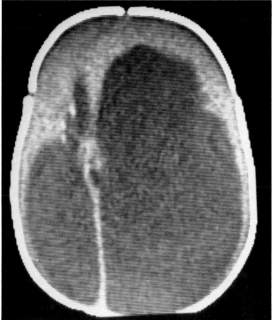

B

FIGURE 7-2. Ventricular septa can develop as sequels to IVH. These are frequently missed by CT. Ultrasound is more sensitive for detection of thin septa, and depicts them routinely. **A**, Septa intersect both lateral ventricles, but are best shown in left lateral ventricle, which is markedly enlarged. **B**, Correlative CT fails to show septa.

periventricular pathology to better advantage, as is discussed later. The roofs of the lateral ventricles are clearly outlined on sonograms, Because of volume averaging in the axial scanning plane, CT does not show this portion of the ventricles in an optimal fashion. Coronal scanning, rarely done in small infants, would be necessary to achieve this. Both CT and ultrasound show ependymal thickening approximately 2–3 weeks after intraventricular hemorrhage. This is ascribed to ependymitis and/or coating with a layer of clotted blood.[23, 24]

With the development of porencephalic cysts in the neonate, the question of ventricular communication between cyst and ventricle may arise. This can present a problem for ultrasound and CT. In both methods, there are difficulties identifying the thin ependyma, which is denuded of its white matter support. However, ultrasound is more likely to recognize a thin layer of tissue, as it shows ventricular septa and septations within porencephalic cysts with greater consistency.

In summary, ventricular size can be easily measured by CT and ultrasound. Under usual clinical conditions, both methods meet expected diagnostic criteria.

Summary Table: Ventricles

Accuracy in depicting size	CT = ultrasound
Advantages of CT	Shows better: Complex ventricular distortion
Advantages of ultrasound	Shows better: Ventricular septa Ependyma and immediate periventricular pathology Communication between ventricles and porencephalic cyst

Intracranial Hemorrhage

- Intracerebral (cerebroventricular) hemorrhage

  Subependymal hemorrhage (SEH)
  Intraventricular hemorrhage (IVH)
  Intraparenchymal hemorrhage (IPH)

- Extracerebral hemorrhage

  Subarachnoid hemorrhage (SAH)
  Subdural/epidural hematoma (SDH, EDH)

Intracerebral Hemorrhage

The most widely used classification of intracerebral hemorrhage is that of Papile.[25] The lowest grade hemorrhage is subependymal bleeding (Grade I). Subependymal hemorrhage (SEH) may extend into the normal-sized ventricular system (Grade II) or cause ventricular dilatation (Grade III). When SEH extends into neighboring brain tissue, the highest degree of hemorrhage is reached (Grade IV).

It was pointed out earlier that germinal matrix-related hemorrhage (SEH, IVH, IPH) is the most prevalent form of cerebral pathology, with an incidence of 43–86% in autopsy series and 40–60% in neonatal survivors. The implications relative to immediate survival and neurodevelopmental handicap were stressed earlier.

Subependymal Hemorrhage (SEH)

SEH is the most common form of intracerebral hemorrhage. It is prevalent among prematures,[5, 26, 27, 29–31] but can also be seen in full-term neonates.[27, 32–34] It occurs as isolated pathology or in association with IVH, and is bilateral in 90%.

In normal neonates, increased echogenicity and density of caudate nuclei may cause false-positive interpretation by ultrasound and CT, respectively. The subependymal germinal matrix consists of tightly packed cells,[4] and this is responsible for the increased density/echogenicity. Another source of confusion and misinterpretation is an anatomic characteristic of the subependymal germinal layer in prematures (up to the gestational age of 30 weeks). In these infants, the germinal matrix follows the lateral ventricle into far-posterior regions. In the case of SEH, the posterior extension of the clot may simulate IVH as material with increased density/echogenicity indents or compresses the lateral ventricles. In our experience, this has been more of a problem for ultrasound than for CT (Fig. 7-3). The axial CT image displays a large segment of the lateral ventricles, and usually shows the smooth medial demarcation of the clot as well as the slitlike residual of the compressed ventricle.

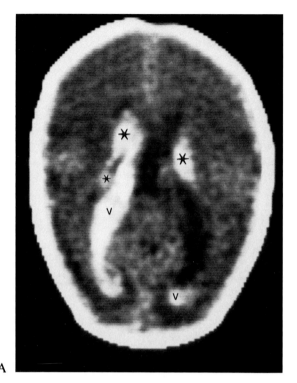

A

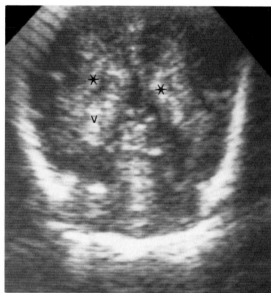

B

FIGURE 7-3. Subependymal versus intraventricular hemorrhage (IVH). Sonograms may not resolve subependymal hemorrhage (SEH) from IVH, particularly when SEH extends posteriorly along the body and tail of the caudate nucleus. **A,** CT shows bilateral SEH (*asterisk*) with moderate posterior extension on right. Associated IVH (*V*), bilaterally, with large blood clot on right. **B,** Correlative sonogram resolves SEH (*asterisk*) and IVH (*V*) less convincingly.

Both ultrasound and CT can miss SEH. The missed diagnosis of a small SEH may not be of far-reaching clinical significance. While the dual application of CT and ultrasound may salvage some cases with a missed diagnosis of SEH, it appears not efficacious to choose this approach. In the case of diagnostic uncertainty, sonography offers the advantage of ease of performance. Follow-up scans may clarify the issue. In the case of true SEH, one may later recognize changes of the germinal matrix echo texture or the evolution of ventricular hemorrhage and/or dilatation.

Summary Table: Subependymal Hemorrhage

Overall accuracy	CT = ultrasound but both modalities miss small hemorrhages. Complementary use of both methods increases accuracy.
General considerations	Ultrasound more practical modality in spite of occasional misdiagnoses.

Intraventricular Hemorrhage (IVH)

The incidence of IVH[2, 4, 6, 18] in neonatal autopsies is 28–73%, slightly less than that of SEH in all reported series. This would appear logical, since not all SEHs rupture into the ventricular system.

IVH is infrequently misdiagnosed by CT. In Ludwig et al.'s series,[6] CT diagnosed all IVHs. In Flodmark et al.'s material,[2] CT produced a few false-positive and false-negative diagnoses. Sonography appears to have a tendency to overcall IVH, while CT is showing a trend toward false-negatives. False-positive diagnoses by ultrasound could be explained on the basis of choroid plexi simulating hemorrhage in small ventricles or the occasional difficulty in sonography in differentiating between intra- and extraventricular hemorrhages. The reduced sensitivity of CT should be related to its inability to depict old blood in the ventricles. As the initial ventricular blood cast retracts and breaks up into multiple small chunks surrounded by CSF, and as these clots become autolyzed, CT may fail to recognize hemorrhage (Fig. 7-4). In contrast, ultrasound is sensitive to these material changes and can image blood even in the later stages of IVH.

Both CT and ultrasound can show ependymal thickening following IVH (Fig. 7-4). This is ascribed to chemical ependymitis and/or coating with clotted blood.[23, 24] Since sequential ultrasound is performed more frequently, this is seen more routinely on sonograms.[28]

Choroid plexus hemorrhage has been reported as a rare source of bleeding in 3–7% of IVH.[2, 18, 35–37] Reeder et al.[34] claimed a 59% incidence, and described sonographic criteria that suggest that diagnosis. We find that the diagnosis of choroid plexus hemorrhage is difficult to make both with CT and sonography.

If one accepts ultrasound's lack of perfect specificity and CT's occasional failure to recognize small intraventricular bleeds, then it would appear appropriate to select ultrasound as the more ideal screening tool for IVH. Ultrasound may overcall some intraventricular hemorrhages, but is less likely to overlook the presence of IVH.

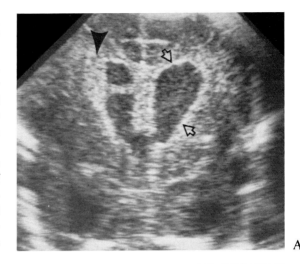

A

Summary Table: Intraventricular Hemorrhage

Overall accuracy	CT = ultrasound Ultrasound has trend toward false-positives. CT has trend toward false-negatives. Complimentary use increases accuracy.
Advantages of ultrasound	Sees blood clots and old blood to better advantage.
General considerations	Ultrasound more practical modality in spite of occasional misdiagnoses.

Intraparenchymal Hemorrhage (IPH)

Intraparenchymal lesions occur in the cortex and white matter of brain and cerebellum. They can represent hemorrhagic infarcts, hemorrhage into zones of periventricular leukencephalopathy, or direct extension from SEH.[4] IPH is less frequent than other types of intracranial hemorrhages; postmortem series sug-

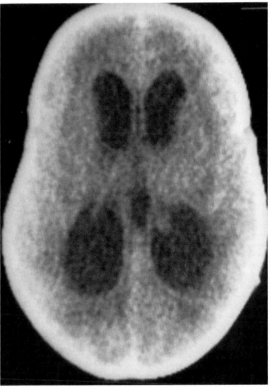

B

FIGURE 7-4. Old intraventricular blood, ventriculitis, ependymitis. This patient had previous IVH. An intraventricular blood clot later disintegrated into larger, then smaller chunks. In addition, klebsiella ventriculitis developed. **A,** Diffusely dispersed midlevel echoes in ventricles represent mixture of old blood and infected CSF. Ependymal thickening (*open arrows*) and periventricular edema (*arrowhead*) are both characterized by high-level echoes. **B,** Corresponding CT shows ventricular enlargement but fails to reveal changes within and outside ventricles.

gest an incidence of 19–24%.[2, 3, 6, 18] It is significantly less common in surviving infants.

In Papile's classification, IPH is considered an extension of SEH into neighboring brain tissue and therefore implies an underlying germinal matrix bleed. While this mechanism may apply for some, Flodmark et al.[2] and Armstrong[7] never observed extension of SEH into brain parenchyma. Flodmark stated that intraparenchymal bleeds almost always represent secondary hemorrhages into white matter. IPH may also result from reentry of intraventricular blood into white matter via rupture of the ventricular wall.[6, 18] Intraparenchymal cerebellar hemorrhage (ICH) is much less common, ranging between 6 and 17%.[2, 4, 6]

The ability of CT to detect ICH in neonates is well documented.[38–47] Similarly, sonography has proven itself in diagnosing intracerebral hemorrhage[48, 49] (Fig. 7-5). The literature suggests good correlation between CT and ultrasound.[48, 50–54] However, the overall diagnostic accuracy of CT appears less for IPH than for other types of intracerebral hemorrhage, for example, SEH and IVH.[2] In Flodmark's autopsy series,[2] there were six false-negative diagnoses and one false-positive.

The literature refers to a high degree of sensitivity and specificity for sonography.[55–57] Sauerbrei et al. reported a false-negative rate of only 4%,[36] while the correlative investigation of Babcock et al.[54] revealed a sensitivity of 100% and a specificity of 94%. In our experience, there is more disagreement between CT and ultrasound on IPH than is suggested in the literature. It is difficult to differentiate nonhemorrhagic periventricular leukomalacia from the hemorrhagic form (Fig. 7-6). Both create increased echogenicity around the ventricles that is similar or identical. Lesions in the occipital area or in the hemispheric cortex may go undetected by ultrasound. The metamorphosis of intracerebral clots from solid, well-circumscribed zones with densely packed high-level echoes to thin-walled porencephalic cysts is well-documented by ultrasound. CT can miss small isodense hematoma, but will detect the evolving porencephalic cyst with ease.

Posterior fossa hemorrhages are difficult to detect both with CT and with ultrasound. This reflects the typically small size of these lesions,[2] but also ultrasound's and CT's inherent limitations of resolving pathologies in the posterior fossa.

This discussion demonstrates that ultrasound and CT are accurate in depicting IPH. However, to obtain perfect diagnostic information, one would need to employ both, a very impractical and costly approach. It appears sensible to use ultrasound in the course of initial investigation and add CT if sonographic findings do not fit the clinical setting or if diagnostic questions arise on the sonogram.

Summary Table:
Intraparenchymal Hemorrhage

Overall accuracy	CT ≧ ultrasound
Advantages of CT	Shows better: High hemispheric hematoma Hematoma in posterior fossa Differentiates more reliably than sonography between periventricular edema and periventricular hemorrhage
General considerations	Ultrasound more practical modality

Extracerebral Hemorrhage

Subarachnoid Hemorrhage (SAH)

SAH is most frequently observed over the hemispheric convexities and in the region of the temporal and occipital lobes.[4] SAH can result from spillage of intraventricular blood into the subarachnoid space via the outlet of the fourth ventricle. Primary SAH may have its cause in hypoxia,[59] ruptured bridging veins and leptomeningeal vessels,[4, 60] or in coagulopathy.[61]

Secondary SAH occurs almost routinely in patients with intraventricular hemorrhage.[2, 6] The literature quotes the incidence of primary SAH in neonatal autopsies to be in the range 9–64%.[2, 6, 18] Ultrasound may recognize SAH as increased echogenicity and as thickened vessels within the cisterns[9] (Fig. 7-5), but low specificity and sensitivity make the modality extremely

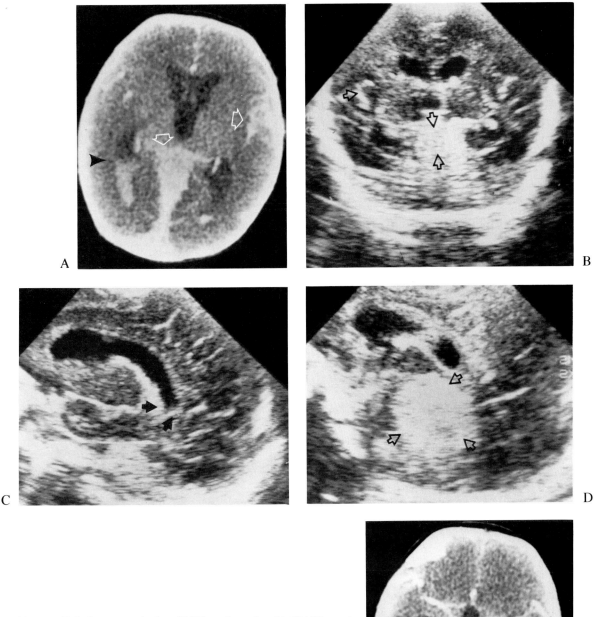

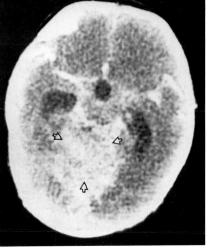

FIGURE 7-5. Intraventricular (IVH), subarachnoid (SAH), and intraparenchymal hemorrhage (IPH) exhibited in a premature infant with coagulopathy. **A**, SAH (*open arrow*) and IVH (*black arrowhead*) are well demonstrated on CT. **B**, SAH also suggested on sonogram by high-level echoes in sylvian, ambient, and supravermian cisterns (*open arrows*). These spaces show high echogenicity in normals. Therefore, this sonographic finding is unreliable for diagnosis of SAH. **C**, Sonogram clearly shows layering of intraventricular blood in temporal horn (*arrows*). IPH in brain stem (*open arrows*), well illustrated on sonogram (**D**) and CT (**E**).

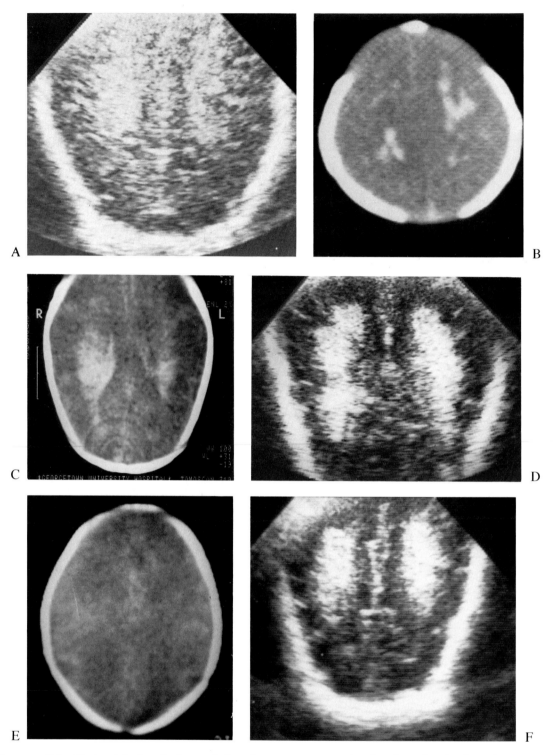

FIGURE 7-6. Periventricular leukencephalopathy (PVL) can present in a hemorrhagic or nonhemorrhagic form. Both subentities result in increased periventricular echodensity. Hemorrhagic foci may submerge within affected zones. **A, B**; Hemorrhagic PVL. Sonogram (**A**) shows diffuse increase of periventricular echogenicity. Focal hemorrhages are not suggested. CT (**B**) identifies hemorrhagic foci in centrum semiovale. Associated edema is not convincingly demonstrated. **C, D**; Hemorrhagic PVL. CT (**C**) shows periventricular and intraventricular hemorrhage. Corresponding sonogram (**D**) shows large diffuse zones of increased echogenicity. **E, F**; nonhemorrhagic PVL. CT (**E**) revealing no hemorrhage on this high axial cut. Sonogram (**F**) with dense echoes in centrum semiovale.

unreliable.[9, 18] CT is hampered by similar shortcomings; SAH over the cerebral convexities is frequently missed.[6] False-positive diagnoses may occur when increased density in the region of falx and interhemispheric fissure is interpreted as SAH (false falx sign).[26]

Overall, CT is more accurate in the diagnosis of SAH. Babcock placed the accuracy of sonography at 60%, and Flodmark stated that of CT was 66%. Our own data show very little agreement between ultrasound and CT. Usually CT suggests SAH by virtue of increased density of the subarachnoid spaces, while sonography in the same cases missed that pathology entirely.

SAH is considered by some as innocuous, as it has been rarely shown to cause death and as survivors are often normal.[4] In the adult, SAH frequently results in adhesive changes of the subarachnoid spaces with ensuing communicating hydrocephalus. It may also lead to arterial spasm with cerebral ischemia and late cortical atrophy. Long-term effects of SAH in neonates have not been sufficiently studied, and therefore a meaningful conclusion cannot be made. Early recognition of SAH is desirable. Only by detecting all forms and variants of intracranial hemorrhage will one be able to judge the impact on neurodevelopmental outcome. CT is a more precise method to diagnose SAH.

Summary Table:
Subarachnoid Hemorrhage

Overall accuracy	CT $\geqslant$ ultrasound
General considerations	CT definitely superior modality. Ultrasound unreliable in diagnosing SAH.

Subdural Hematoma (SDH)

The overall incidence of subdural hematoma (SDH) varies among authors, and is reported to be in the range 3–18%.[2, 59] Birth trauma plays a major role in its development. Cranial distortion during birth can lead to rupture of bridging veins or to a tear of dural folds. Hypoxia and SDH often coexist,[4] and associated neurologic symptoms may be more reflective of the underlying hypoxia than of SDH.

Because of the near-field artifact, ultrasound is less apt to diagnose frontal subdural hema-

toma (Fig. 7-7). Limitation of near- and far-field resolution and the pieshaped beam configuration make it difficult to optimally investigate pathologies close to the periphery of brain with standard scanning methods. This diminishes the sensitivity of ultrasound for SDH. The use of high-frequency transducers, and coupling devices to be fitted over the cranium, can reduce some of the shortcomings.[12]

While the accuracy of CT for diagnosing small SDHs in neonates has its limitations,[2] CT has a much greater chance of identifying extracerebral fluid collections as compared to ultrasound.

Summary Table: Subdural Hematoma

Overall accuracy	CT $\geqslant$ ultrasound
General considerations	Because of near-field artifact and suboptimal visualization of brain periphery, ultrasound may miss SDHs. CT more precise.

Parenchymal Lesions

Nonhemorrhagic ischemic/Hypoxic Changes

    Focal: (Periventricular leukomalacia; cortical infarcts)
    Generalized: (Cerebral edema)

Loss of brain mass

    Atrophy

Nonhemorrhagic Ischemic/Hypoxic Changes

Periventricular Leukomalacia (PVL): Infarcts

The role of nonhemorrhagic ischemic/hypoxic cerebral pathologies relative to late neurodevelopmental outcome and their frequency (7–57%) was stressed earlier. This disease entity is of considerable importance, because it accounts for a large group of neonates that leave the early state of infancy with various forms of cerebral palsy and mental retardation, as well as hearing and visual deficiencies.

This group of pathologies has attracted little

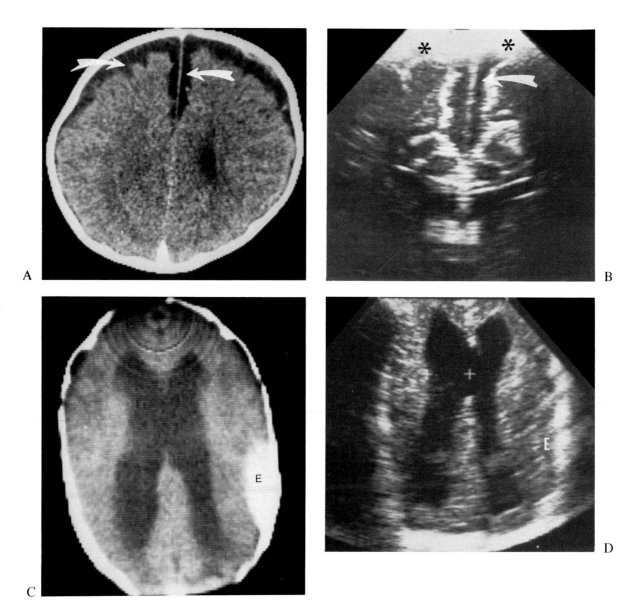

A

B

C

D

FIGURE 7-7. Extracerebral hemorrhage. Epidural or subdural hematoma is difficult to show on sonograms. The echogenicity differential between brain and extracerebral blood may not be sufficient to allow recognition. In frontal areas, near-field artifact and exclusion of parts of brain secondary to triangular beam shape can make diagnosis of extracerebral hematoma difficult or impossible. **A, B**; Subdural hygroma in frontal area, clearly depicted (**A**) on CT (*curved arrows*). Sonogram (**B**) only shows interhemispheric extension of same (*curved arrow*); frontal convexity collection is submerged in dense near-field artifact (*asterisk*). Temporal-parietal epidural hematoma (*E*) on CT (**C**) is missed on sonogram (**D**).

attention in the imaging literature because of the deficiencies of CT and ultrasound in diagnosing this disorder. CT was initially heralded as a competent diagnostic tool in the diagnosis of leukencephalopathies. Later reports retracted the initial CT claims, and emphasized the difficulty of accurately imaging PVL in the neonatal age group.[2, 63-65] The periventricular hypodensity, initially interpreted as periventricular edema or necrosis, was later shown to be normal in most premature and full-term infants.[6, 64, 66] This is caused by increased water content in the infant brain and lack of myelin-ization.[66] Between the physiologic localized periventricular hypodensity in the normal neo-nate and the abnormal generalized hypodensity in diffuse edema lies a spectrum of density changes that leads from the normal to the ab-normal state (Fig. 7-8). While it is difficult to define the exact border between normal and ab-normal, there is a point where the degree of periventricular hypodensity no longer reflects normalcy. Since CT numbers are extremely un-reliable for the infant brain, that judgment must be made on the basis of personal experience and follow-up. In contrast, generalized edema can be reliably diagnosed by CT.[2] In Flod-mark's CT autopsy series,[2] a false diagnosis of ischemic brain damage was made in 32 of 90 diseased neonates. In the same series, general-ized edema was correctly diagnosed in 94%.

In Babcock et al.'s small ultrasound autopsy series,[17] ischemic brain damage was only seen in association with hemorrhage. Other authors share the conviction that focal ischemia cannot be diagnosed by sonography.[9, 12] There is some disagreement on the ultrasound appearance of cerebral edema. Some authors have described edema as anechoic areas surrounding cerebral vessels and gyri[12]; others suggested that cere-bral edema increased echo texture.[58, 74]

Cerebral Edema

We find that cerebral edema is shown as a zone of increased echogenicity (Fig. 7-8). In PVL, this is most pronounced in the periventricular areas, particularly the centrum semiovale and the forceps major and minor. Since the degree of echogenicity cannot be measured in absolute terms, it is difficult to determine exactly which echo density denotes edema. It is therefore left to the examiner's experience and in judgment to determine whether the periventricular echo-genicity has passed the threshhold of normalcy. While PVL may be difficult to diagnose in its early stage, which is dominated by edema, the more advanced stages are easily recognized with ultrasound. These later stages are charac-terized by the development of periventricular cysts. We have reported this white matter cavi-tation in 21 patients and referred to it as cystic periventricular leukencephalopathy.[73]

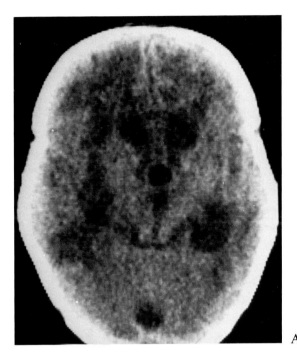

A

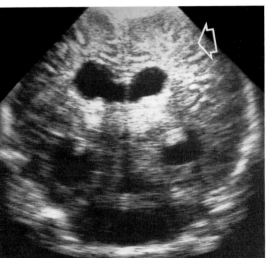

B

FIGURE 7-8. Edema. White matter edema can result from hemorrhagic and nonhemorrhagic leukencepha-lopathy, but can also be associated with encephalitis. CT (**A**) and sonogram (**B**) of premature infant with periventricular leukencephalopathy (PVL) show periventricular hypodensity on CT (**A**), particularly in frontal area. This can be difficult to interpret be-cause of normal occurrence in neonates and young infants. **B**, Increased periventricular echogenicity is seen on sonogram (*arrow*), following geographic dis-tribution of white matter. This is a reliable sono-graphic sign of edema.

CT is less accurate in depicting small periventricular cysts, probably because of density averaging. It was previously mentioned that the multidirectional sonographic scanning shows the ventricular perimeter to better advantage. Since most of the cysts are aligned in a semicircular fashion around the lateral ventricles, they are better imaged on ultrasound. In the older infant with decreasing accessibility of the anterior fontanelle, CT becomes the better method for showing cystic PVL.

We believe that cystic PVL represents but an extreme form of PVL that is characterized by tissue necrosis. It is important to start recognizing the lesser, reversible forms of PVL, because this may have therapeutic and prognostic consequences. In the beginning of this chapter, we referred to a group of handicapped infants who had no documentable cerebral abnormalities or only Grade I intracerebral hemorrhage. This is an interesting category of patients. One could theorize that this group of patients may have suffered the lesser, noncystic form of PVL that went unrecognized by CT and ultrasound.

We have pointed out that both sonography and CT can identify nonhemorrhagic ischemic brain pathologies by increased echogenicity or decreased tissue attenuation. We also stressed the potential diagnostic dilemmas for CT and ultrasound as well as the advantages of sonography in recognizing small cysts. CT has a definitive advantage over ultrasound as far as tissue typification is concerned. For example, in the case of partially hemorrhagic PVL, ultrasound cannot differentiate between hemorrhagic and edematous tissue, whereas CT has no difficulty in making that distinction.[10] Smaller ischemic changes may be undiagnosable by ultrasound. In our experience CT is more accurate under these circumstances. However, both CT and ultrasound usually miss tiny foci of necrosis. If strategically located, these small pathologies can cause major neurologic deficits without being traceable on CT and ultrasound.

Summary Table:
Periventricular Leukencephalopathy

Overall accuracy	Ultrasound ≫ CT
Advantages of ultrasound	Ultrasound shows better: Periventricular edema Periventricular cysts
Advantages of CT	CT distinguishes better between hemorrhagic and nonhemorrhagic PVL.

Atrophy

Cerebral and/or cerebellar atrophy can have many causes. Atrophy can signify irreversible brain damage with very poor prognosis.[67, 68] Patients with cerebral atrophy show a high incidence of neurodevelopmental handicap.[1] The limitations of ultrasound for imaging the brain convexity and the areas close to the inner table of the calvarium were discussed earlier. However, the introduction of 7.5-MHz transducers and computer-assisted sonography have added a new dimension to sonographic imaging of brain close to the anterior fontanelle. The subfrontal and interhemispheric subarachnoid spaces are now much more clearly outlined, and atrophy can be more easily diagnosed. CT represents the superior modality for diagnosing atrophy, as it depicts surface morphology more completely and more accurately.

Summary Table: Atrophy

Overall accuracy	CT > ultrasound
Advantages of CT	Shows/gives better global view of brain surface, whereas sonography sees preferentially frontal region with interhemispheric fissure. More accurate assessment of atrophy with CT.

Miscellaneous Anatomic Structures and Pathologies

Calvarium

Evaluation of the calvarium should be part of a neurodiagnostic evaluation of the central nervous system (CNS). In congenital anomalies, skull defects can give a clue to the nature of the abnormality. Dysplastic changes of the calvarium can be seen with Arnold–Chiari malformations (Lueckenschaedel) and bone defects of variable size are part of encephaloceles. Large skull defects can be discerned by ultrasound, but smaller abnormalities are not seen. CT allows detailed analysis of the skull and is the preferred diagnostic tool.

Vascular Structures

Real-time sonography has the unique capability of observing vascular pulsation. The usage of intravenous contrast material with CT provides a superior modus for stationary evaluation of cerebral vasculature. Small vascular abnormalities cannot be reliably diagnosed with either method, and arteriography is needed for definitive diagnosis. Large vascular abnormalities such as vein of Galen aneurysms can be recognized with both methods, but smaller ones are better demonstrated with CT.

Intracranial Calcifications

CT and sonography are extremely sensitive to high-density changes within the brain. With ultrasound, calcifications show as focal areas of high echogenicity. Unfortunately, shadowing behind the calcification may be difficult to elicit. CT demarcates the abnormalities as high-attenuation foci (Fig. 7-9). Both methods have similar potential.[74]

Computed Tomography versus Sonography: Other Considerations Concerning Choice of Modality

In previous sections, we compared two competing diagnostic modalities. Here, we wish to concentrate on the practical advantages and disadvantages of each method.

The advantages of ultrasound are quite obvious and in many respects overwhelming, particularly if one considers lower cost, lack of potential radiation risk, limited patient handling, and

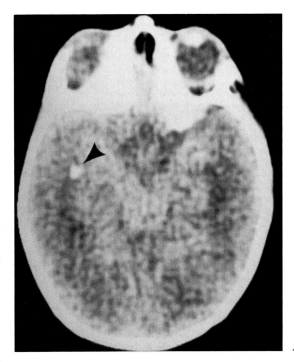

A

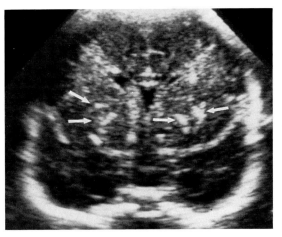

B

FIGURE 7-9. Calcifications. Patient with congenital parenchymal calcification, presumably secondary to toxoplasmosis. **A**, A single focus of calcium is shown on CT (*arrowhead*). **B**, Coronal sonographic cut shows coarse accumulation of high-level echoes in both basal ganglia (*arrows*) without sonographic shadowing. The full extent of basal ganglia calcification is missed by CT, probably because of partial volume averaging. Both CT and ultrasound are sensitive to recognition of parenchymal calcium. It must be understood, however, that observed cerebral calcifications rarely produce sonographic shadowing. Foci of dense echoes therefore must alert observer for possible presence of calcium. CT is needed for definitive diagnosis.

reduced disruption of the protective milieu. From this point of view, the choice of modality is heavily in favor of sonography.

Advances in neonatal intensive care and the notoriety of anoxia/ischemia in this patient group call for a diagnostic method that can portray cerebral pathology with a high degree of accuracy—a method whose frequent and repetitive use is not prohibitive in terms of cost and radiation exposure. Ultrasound, therefore, appears particularly suited for screening. Since many CNS changes in the neonatal age group are subclinical and may escape clinical recognition, it becomes increasingly important to recognize brain abnormalities through routine testing of all neonates at risk. (Proposed screening schedules are discussed elsewhere.) While ultrasound has many advantages over CT, there is also a definitive role for CT. In the older infant, the choice of technique begins to favor CT, since the anterior fontanelle becomes increasingly less accessible for ultrasound. After the eighteenth month of life, the anterior fontanelle is usually closed unless increased intracranial pressure exists that may keep it open. While transcalvarial scanning is possible, the image quality tends to suffer.

When the sonographic findings are not compatible with the clinical setting, a CT scan should be performed. CT may add diagnostic information in cases of questionable intracerebral hemorrhage. CT may depict peripherally located intracerebral hematoma, subarachnoid hemorrhage, atrophy, or unsuspected subdural collections. Nonhemorrhagic ischemic changes may be more obvious on CT or may require dual imaging because of insufficient information from either method. The complex anatomic changes associated with congenital anomalies usually become more apparent with CT scanning; there is no image degradation in near- and far-field and all parts of the anatomic slice are clearly visualized. Most ultrasound examinations do not include the anterolateral margins of the brain because of the triangular or square configuration of the ultrasound beam. Also, quality and completeness of a sonogram is determined by operator skill and knowledge of the site of suspected pathology. CT provides a complete anatomic cross section, and is not operator dependent.

Further refinement of neonatal care may call for increased precision of the diagnostic process. This is particularly true for nonhemorrhagic ischemic changes, such as leukomalacia and infarcts. In this setting, the use of both modalities may be invaluable. It is suggested by some that ultrasound be used for the preterm infant while CT is reserved for the term infant. We believe that the selection of diagnostic modality should be made on the basis of diagnostic propriety and not on infant maturity. The advantages and limitations of ultrasound and CT are valid for both premature and mature babies.

References

1. Stewart AL, Thornburn RJ, Hope PL, Goldsmith M, Reynolds EOR, Lipscomb AP. Relation between ultrasound appearance of the brain in very preterm infants and neurodevelopmental outcome at 18 months of age. In: The Second Special Ross Laboratories Conference on Perinatal Intracranial Hemorrhage, Syllabus, 1090–1116, 1982.
2. Flodmark O, Becker LE, Harwood-Nash DC, Fitzhardinge PM, Fitz CR, Chuang SH. Correlation between computed tomography and autopsy in premature and full-term neonates that have suffered perinatal asphyxia. Radiology 137:93–103, 1980.
3. Bozynski ME, Nelson MN, Genaze DR, Chilcote RG, Ramsey RG, Clasen RA, O'Donnell KJ, Meier WA. Longitudinal follow-up by ultrasound of intracranial hemorrhage and ventriculomegaly in relation to developmental outcome in infants weighing <1,200 grams at birth. In: The Second Special Ross Laboratories Conference on Perinatal Intracranial Hemorrhage, Syllabus, 1153–1175, 1982.
4. Pape KE, Wigglesworth JS. Hemorrhage, ischemia and the perinatal brain. In: Clinics in Developmental Medicine, Numbers 69/70, Pape KE, Wigglesworth HS, eds. London, William Heinemann/Philadelphia, Lippincott, 1979.
5. Leech RW, Kohnen P. Subependymal and intraventricular hemorrhages in the newborn. Am J Pathol 77:465–476, 1974.
6. Ludwig B, Becker K, Rutter G, Bohl J, Brand M. Postmortem CT and autopsy in perinatal intracranial hemorrhage. AJNR 4:27–36, 1983.
7. Armstrong DD. Intraventricular hemorrhage. Pathology of short-term survivors. In: The Second Special Ross Laboratories Conference on Perina-

tal Intracranial Hemorrhage, Syllabus, 1074–1089, 1982.

8. Shinnar S, Molteni RA, Gammon K, D'Souza BJ, Altman J, Freeman JM. Intraventricular hemorrhage in the premature infant. A changing outlook. N Engl J Med 306:1464–1486, 1982.

9. Rumack CM, Johnson ML. Neonatal brain imaging: choosing between modalities. Diagn Imaging 28–33, 1983.

10. Shankaran S, Slovis TL, Bedard MP, Bedard MP, Poland RL. Sonographic classification of intracranial hemorrhage. A prognostic indication of mortality, morbidity and short-term neurologic outcome. J Pediatr 100:469, 1982.

11. Fleischer AC, Hutchison AA, Kirchner SG, James AE. Cranial sonography of the preterm neonate. Diagn Imaging 2011, 1981.

12. Ment LR, Scott DT, Rothman SG, Ehrenkranz RS, Warshaw JB. Neurodevelopmental follow-up of VLBW neonates: effects of GMH/IVH (abstr). Pediatr Res 15:1592, 1981.

13. Schechner S, Ross G, Auld P. Early neurodevelopmental outcome of low-birth-weight infants surviving neonatal intraventricular hemorrhage. In: Perinatal intracranial hemorrhage, Ross Laboratories Conference, Washington, D.C., Syllabus, 724–735, 1980.

14. Papile LA, Burstein J, Burstein R, Koffler H, Koops BL, Johnson JD. Posthemorrhagic hydrocephalus in low-birthweight infants: treatment by serial lumbar punctures. J Pediatr 97:273–277, 1980.

15. Krishnamoorthy KS, Todres ID, Kuehnle KJ, Shannon DC, DeLong GR, Davis KR. Neurologic sequelae in the survivors of neonatal intraventricular hemorrhage. In: Perinatal intracranial hemorrhage, Ross Laboratories Conference, Washington, D.C., Syllabus, 697–710, 1980.

16. Stewart AL, Reynolds EOR, Lipscomb AP. Outcome for infants of very low-birthweight: survey of the world literature. Lancet I:1038–1041, 1981.

17. Babcock DS, Bove KE, Han BK. Intracranial hemorrhage in premature infants: sonographic–pathologic correlation. AJNR 3:309–317, 1982.

18. Garret WJ, Kossoff G, Jones RFC. Ultrasonic cross-sectional visualization of hydrocephalus in infants. Neuroradiology 8:279–288, 1975.

19. Lees RF, Harrison RB, Sims TL. Grey scale ultrasonography in the evaluation of hydrocephalus and associated abnormalities in infants. Am J Dis Child 132:376–378, 1978.

20. Skolnick ML, Rosenbaum AE, Matzuk T, Guthkelch AN, Heinz ER. Detection of dilated cerebral ventricles in infants. A correlative study between ultrasound and computed tomography. Radiology 131:447–451, 1979.

21. Morgan CL, Trought WS, Rothman SJ, Jiminez JR. Comparison of gray-scale ultrasonography and computed tomography in the evaluation of macrocrania in infants. Radiology 132:119–123, 1979.

22. James AE, Flor WJ, Novak GR, et al. The ultrastructural basis of periventricular edema: preliminary studies. Radiology 135:747–750, 1980.

23. Sherwood A, Hopp A, Smith JF. Cellular reactions to subependymal hemorrhage in the human neonate. Neuropathol Appl Neurobiol 4:245–261, 1978.

24. Papile LA, Burstein J, Burstein R, Koffler H. Incidence and evolution of subependymal intraventricular hemorrhage: a study of infants with birthweights less than 1500 grams. J Pediatr 92:529–534, 1978.

25. Harcke HT, Naeye RL, Storch A, Blank WA. Perinatal cerebral intraventricular hemorrhage. J Pediatr 80:37–42, 1972.

26. Fedrick J, Butler NR. Certain causes of neonatal death. II. Intraventricular hemorrhage. Biol Neonate 15:257–290, 1970.

27. Reeder JD, Sanders RC. Ventriculitis in the neonate: recognition by sonography. AJNR 4:37–41, 1983.

28. Deonna T, Payot M, Probat A, Probst A, Prodhom LS. Neonatal intracranial hemorrhage in premature infants. Pediatrics 56:1056–1064, 1975.

29. Hambleton G, Wigglesworth JS. Origin of intraventricular hemorrhage in the preterm infant. Arch Dis Child 51:651–659, 1976.

30. Baldes-Dapena MAS, Arey JB. The causes of neonatal mortality: an analysis of 501 autopsies on newborn infants. J Pediatr 77:366–375, 1970.

31. Maki Y, Shirai S. Angiographic findings in intraventricular hemorrhage in newborn infants. Acta Radiol (Suppl) [Stockh] 347:167–174, 1975.

32. Palma PA, Miner ME, Morriss FH. Intraventricular hemorrhage in the neonate born at term. Am J Dis Child 133:941–944, 1979.

33. Friede RL. Residual lesions of infantile cerebral phlebothrombosis. Acta Neuropathol (Berl) 22:319–332, 1972.

34. Reeder JD, Jaude JV, Setzer ES. Choroid plexus hemorrhage in premature neonates: recognition by sonography. AJNR 3:619–622, 1982.

35. Friede R. Developmental Neuropathology. New York, Springer-Verlag, 28, 1975.

36. Sauerbrei EE, Digney M, Harrison PB, Cooperberg PL. Ultrasonic evaluation of neonatal intracranial hemorrhage and its complications. Radiology 139:677–685, 1981.

37. Jacobs L. Kinkel WR, Heffner RR. Autopsy correlation of computerized tomography: experience with 6000 CT scans. Arch Neurol 43:602–607, 1977.

38. Messina AV. Cranial computerized tomography. A radiologic pathologic correlation. Arch Neurol 43:602–607, 1977.

39. Zimmerman RA, Billaniuk LT, Gennarelli T, Bruce D, Dolinskas C, Uzzell B. Cranial computed tomography in diagnosis and management of acute head trauma. AJR 131:27–34, 1978.

40. Burstein J, Papile LA, Burstein R. Intraventricular hemorrhage and hydrocephalus in premature newborns: a prospective study with CT. AJR 132:631–635, 1979.

41. Lee BCP, Grassi AE, Schechner A, Auld PAM. Neonatal intraventricular hemorrhage: a serial computed tomography study. J Comput Assist Tomogr 3:483–490, 1979.

42. Lazzara A, Ahmann P, Dykes F, Brann AW, Schwartz J. Clinical predictability of intraventricular hemorrhage in preterm infants. Pediatrics 65:30–34, 1980.

43. Pevsner PH, Garcia-Bunuel R, Leeds N, Finkelstein M. Subependymal and intraventricular hemorrhage in neonates. early diagnosis by computed tomography. Radiology 119:111–114, 1976.

44. Krishnamoorthy KS, Fernandez RA, Momose KJ, Delong GR, Moyland FMB, Todres JD, Shannon DC. Evaluation of neonatal intracranial hemorrhage by computerized tomography. Pediatrics 59:165–172, 1977.

45. Burstein J, Papile L, Burstein R. Subependymal germinal matrix and intraventricular hemorrhage in premature infants: diagnosis by CT. AJR 128:971–976, 1977.

46. Rumack CM, McDonald MM, O'Meara OW, Sanders BB, Rudikoff JC. CT detection and course of intracranial hemorrhage in premature infants. AJR 131:493–497, 1978.

47. Pape KE, Cusick G, Houang MTW, Blackwell RJ, Sherwood A, Thorburn RJ, Reynolds EOR. Ultrasound detection of brain damage in preterm infants. Lancet I:1261–1264, 1979.

48. Mack LA, Wright K, Hirsch JH, Alford EC, Guthrie RD, Shuman WP, Rogers JV, Bolender NF. Intracranial hemorrhage in premature infants: accuracy of sonographic evaluation. AJR 137:245–250, 1981.

49. London DA, Carroll BA, Enzmann DR. Sonography of ventricular size and germinal matrix hemorrhage in premature infants. AJR 135:559–564, 1980.

50. Grant EG, Schellinger D, Borts FT, McCullough DC, Friedman GR, Sivasubramanian, KN, Smith Y. Real-time sonography of the neonatal and infant head. AJNR 1:487–492, 1980.

51. Sauerbrei EE, Harrision PB, Ling E, Cooperberg PL. Neonatal intracranial pathology demonstrated by high-frequency linear array ultrasound. JCU 9:427–433, 1981.

52. Johnson ML, Rumack CM, Mannes EJ, Appareti KE. Detection of neonatal intracranial hemorrhage utilizing real-time and static ultrasound. JCU 9:427–433, 1981.

53. Silverboard G, Horder MH, Ahmann PA, Lazzara A, Schwartz JF. Reliability of ultrasound in the diagnosis of intracerebral hemorrhage and posthemorrhagic hydrocephalus: comparison with computed tomographic scan. In: Perinatal Intracranial Hemorrhage, Ross Laboratories Conference, Washington, D.C., Syllabus, 501–513, 1980.

54. Babcock D, Han B. The accuracy of high resolution real-time ultrasonography of the head in infancy. Radiology 139:665–676, 1981.

55. Grant EG, Borts F, Schellinger D, McCullough D, Sivasubramanian KN, Smith, Y. Real-time ultrasonography of neonatal intraventricular hemorrhage and comparison with computed tomography. Radiology 139:685–689, 1981.

56. Pape K, Bennett-Britton S, Syzmonowicz W, Martin D, Fitz C, Becker L. Diagnostic accuracy of neonatal brain imaging: a postmortem correlation. Pediatr Res 15:1597, 1981 (abstr).

57. Martin DC, Hill A, Daneman A, Fitz CR, Becker LE. Focal hypoxic/ischemic cerebral injury in the neonatal brain: sonographic features with computed tomography correlation. In: The Second Special Ross Laboratories Conference on Intracranial Hemorrhage, Syllabus, 513–526, 1982.

58. Larroche JC. Developmental Pathology of the Neonate. Amsterdam, Excerpta Medica, 1977.

59. Towbin A. Central nervous system damage in the human fetus and newborn infant. Mechanical and hypoxic injury incurred in the fetal-neonatal period. Am J Dis Child 119:529–542, 1970.

60. Chessels JM, Wigglesworth JS. Secondary haemorrhagic disease of the newborn. Arch Dis Child 45:539–543, 1970.

61. Osborn AG, Anderson RE, Wing SD. The false falx sign. Radiology 134:421–425, 1980.

62. Albright L, Fellows R. Sequential CT scanning after neonatal intracerebral hemorrhage. AJR 136:949–953, 1981.

63. Estrada M, El Gammal T, Dyken PR. Periventricular low attenuation. A normal finding in computerized tomographic scans of neonates? Arch Neurol 37:754–756, 1980.

64. Schrumpf JD, Sehring S, Killpack S, Brady JP, Hirata T, Mednick JP. Correlation of early neu-

rologic outcome and CT findings in neonatal brain hypoxia and injury. J Comput Assist Tomogr 4:445–450, 1980.

65. Quencer RM. Maturation of normal primate white matter: computed tomographic correlation. AJR 139:561–568, 1982.

66. Armstrong D, Norman M. Periventricular leukomalacia in neonates. Complications and sequelae. Arch Dis Child 49:367–375, 1974.

67. Volpe JJ. Cited at the Perinatal Intracranial Hemorrhage, Ross Laboratories Conference, Washington, D.C., 1980.

68. Leech RW, Alford EC. Morphologic variations in periventricular leukomalacia. Am J Pathol 74:591–600, 1974.

69. Armstrong D, Norman MG. Periventricular leukomalacia in neonates. Complications and sequelae. Arch Dis Child 49:367–375, 1974.

70. Shuman RM, Selednik LH. Periventricular leukomalacia. A One-Year Autopsy Study. Neurology 37:231–235, 1980.

71. Banker BQ, Larroche JC. Periventricular leukomalacia of infancy. Arch Neurol 7:386–410, 1962.

72. Schellinger D, Grant EG, Richardson JD. Cystic periventricular leukomalacia: sonographic and CT findings. AJNR 5:439–445, 1984.

73. Babcock DS, Ball W. Ultrasound diagnosis and short-term prognosis of post-asphyxial encephalopathy in term infants. In: The Second Special Ross Laboratories Conference on Intracranial Hemorrhage, Syllabus, 697–721, 1982.

74. Grant EG, Williams AL, Schellinger D, Slovis T. Intracranial calcification in the infant and neonate: evaluation by sonography and CT. Radiology 1985; 157:63–68.

Index